the cannabis doula

the transparent enlightenment
of my own rebirth

melanin ajé seshat

First Edition, 2020
ISBN 978-0-578-80539-9
Melanin & Books
Washington D.C.
www.thecannabisdoula.com

Information contained within this book is not intended to replace any
medical advice or childbirth education. If you are considering consuming cannabis during pregnancy, or while nursing, please consult
with your primary care provider and a qualified cannabis practitioner.

for Black girls who never made it out
of the box that society places us in

for my sistagirl,
soul sista, and roomies

for mamas
& for all mama's babies

For my hero,
Toni Morrison,
who said we must write

contents

She does not know her beauty
She thinks her brown body has no glory
If she could dance naked under palm trees and see her image in the river
she would know but there are no palm trees on the streets
and dishwater gives back no images.

-William Waring Cuney

Introduction

I'm writing this because I've lived it. The information I'm sharing here is deeply personal, intimate, and sacred knowledge. Knowledge that I've acquired from ten years of using cannabis, both recreationally and medicinally. This is sacred knowledge imparted to me by my ancestors. By wise people who came before me, people who've cultivated this sacred plant, sold it, and made use of it in many ways through unsurmountable odds. The cannabis plant that we know and consume today was used by our ancestors for sacred spiritual traditions and medicinal purposes in Africa, and survived the brutality of chattel slavery where it spread to cultures all over North and South America through what was known as the Transatlantic Slave Trade. These are our traditions. I honor them. I deeply believe that supplementing with cannabis to address endocannabinoid deficiencies in Black women can heal the multitude of physical, mental, and emotional issues that we experience. Cannabis can aid in the holistic healing of our community—the collective healing of the mind, body, and spirit of Black people.

Through The Cannabis Doula, I share my personal and intimate experiences consuming cannabis, evidence-based information and research on cannabis use for a variety of female health concerns, including pregnancy, childbirth, and postpartum, some remedies, tips, and experiences of some of the women I've met along this journey of holistically healing myself with cannabis.

For so long, women have been forced to conceal our cannabis consumption. Due to cannabis prohibition, propaganda and criminalization brought on by the war on drugs, Black women and families have especially suffered from mis-education and stigma surrounding this miraculous plant. I hope that my story, and this book, changes your perception of cannabis. I pray that you use this information to make bold changes in your life, and in the lives of others. Let's Shatter the Stigma.

It's only right that I start by telling you where I come from and how I got here. All of these things have, in some way, impacted my use and knowledge of the cannabis plant. Wouldn't you want to know what inspired all of this? I was born in Chicago, Illinois. My parents are no strangers to marijuana. My dad was a big reefer-head back in his day, as he tells it. We've shared some of thee best conversations on weed. He even detailed his experience before ses became popular, a time when cannabis seeds would put holes in his pockets. My mom, on the other hand, has very negative attitudes about marijuana. She detests it. I went to visit her one weekend in college and she found an old roach in my car and said that it "reeked" of weed. She was horrified! I laughed it off. Literally laughed at my mom. You can imagine how heated she was. Nonetheless, she now blames me for having introduced my older sister and younger brother to smoking it. I told her she should be thanking me! I truly mean it.

I wasn't always this confident in my cannabis consumption, or even the true medicinal benefits of cannabis. In college, when I first started smoking I was slapped regularly in the face with a ton of bricks full of stigma and shame. Apparently, women didn't smoke weed. Or should I say, a lady doesn't smoke weed. As a woman loving weed, it gave me this added mystery and allure. It was appealing to men, who especially reinforced this stereotype saying things like, "I don't date women who smoke weed," or "its unattractive" —as they rolled the biggest blunt and passed it to me. They wouldn't date me, they'd said, but the sex was always out of this world. I figured, they just didn't have enough money to buy weed for the both of us. Looking back on my college days, I realized there are three types of college girls. The ones who drink and the ones who smoke, and the ones who do both, a lot. I've been all three. Interestingly, it's the girls who smoke that seem to peek the interest of men in deeply intimate ways. I think cannabis is a bridge from the male mind to the female mind; as if only under the consumption of cannabis can we truly relate and be vulnerable with one another.

Prior to using cannabis as a superpower, I was hypnotized by the cannabis stigma. I even fell victim to it by judging other women for smoking too much, or subjecting myself to the silly idea that women shouldn't buy weed, let alone sell it. At the same time, I was also consuming a lot of alcohol. A bottle of wine a week was a goal and celebration for me. I mean, weed had to be illegal for a reason, right? Binge drinking in college, from Thursday to Sunday was the norm for many of us. I admired the women who smoked freely, like my roommate, who I always admired for her love of weed regardless of what anyone else had to say about it.

I used to talk to a boy in high school who was the biggest weedhead. When I tell you, this guy would come to school high as a fucking kite. Eyes red as hell. And guess what—I adored him. He was the most amazing, funny, ridiculously charming guy I'd ever met. He was my first real crush and my biggest crush at the time. He loved weed. And he didn't care who knew, how much he smelled like it, he was Scooter and he was gone smoke regardless. I can still taste the weed and pizza in his breath from my first kiss. Funny thing though, he never introduced me to weed. He never forced me to smoke or even mentioned it. I didn't even entertain the thought of smoking until college, but I always knew he smoked. I was the naive cheerleader; the good girl who thought I could get a bad boy, the star of the football team, to stop smoking.

Years later, when I first started smoking, I finally understood why he'd smoke before school, and after, and anytime he wanted. I finally understood why he was so free with his marijuana use, and why he didn't care what anyone had to say. It took me ten years to gain the confidence in cannabis that Scooter had from the jump! When I have the chance to breed a very sedating broad leaf strain of marijuana that makes you laugh so hard you cry, I would name it Scooter in his honor. It would be the dankest, most pungent weed possible. I'm thankful for his life, and his confidence in his own cannabis consumption.

Shattering the Stigma in our lives take work! It takes education. When I decided to start smoking cannabis and really enjoy it, I did a lot of research. I learned about the history of the plant and when it started to be considered illegal. I learned about the War on Drugs and about racism. I read *The New Jim Crow*. I realized there was more to be told. I started asking questions. First, I'd ask my weedman about the names of the strains and where they got it from. They rarely knew what they were selling but always said it came from California, or they would refuse to tell me and ask if I was the feds. There was only one weedman that I can remember who knew as much about weed as I did at the time. Many people didn't even know that it was a plant...let alone a flower. Education is a powerful tool. When I was educated enough on the benefits of cannabis, I was comfortable enough to consume it with my brother. There was no way I was going to be held responsible for introducing my siblings to anything dangerous and addictive—that's just not me. I know better. When I was using cannabis regularly in college, I was able to slow down on the binge drinking that had become a normal part of college, and I was able to make better decisions. I made the Dean's List during each of the three semesters that I heavily consumed cannabis. I was the Chapter President of my sorority and held plenty leadership roles on campus and off campus. But the stigma was always there.

During my senior year of college, I was also leading a drug and alcohol prevention group for teens as an internship at a local nonprofit. Many of them were there because for smoking marijuana. I think about the teens I supported, and even Scooter back in high school, and some of the experience of my friends during that time, and I can't help but think of how beneficial holistic cannabis consumption and education can be in supporting teens during some of the hardest times of their lives. Instead, we give them things like adderall and antidepressants, and they self-medicate with alcohol and whatever prescription drug they can find. They mimic our behavior. Once we develop healthy attitudes toward cannabis, youth will also. As families, the healing that will take place from that is truly dynamic and world changing.

Next, I spent a lot of time talking to elders about cannabis. Their experiences are also important in understanding just how different cannabis is now, versus what they were consuming back in their day. After moving from my hometown of Chicago to Washington DC in 2014, I decided I was going to smoke whenever I wanted and be proud. Here, is where I fell in love with cannabis. I was introduced to this really cool weedman, who knew so much about keeping good weed. An OG. He knew the names of the strains that he was selling and was very experienced. I felt safe. I trusted him and his product. I fell in love with weed, and we would never part from then on. I smoked all the time. In public, in parks, walking to the metro. I always smelled like weed. I would ride the metro with thee loudest weed in my purse, and laugh at people's reaction as I walked pass. I love a good sesh. A sesh is when you gather with friends and smoke weed, usually with food, music, and intellectual conversation. I was happy to talk to people about it and always eager to smoke, even if I couldn't always afford to put on or match, I would always offer to roll up.

However, not being fully knowledgeable about cannabis can lead to dangerous situations. It definitely landed me in some uncomfortable situations with fake people, in college and after. I was often very naive in my cannabis consumption, relying on men to provide the flower, which is never safe. I hope that from my experience, women will feel more comfortable buying or growing their own cannabis, knowing what's quality, and knowing what is safe to consume.

I've heard stories of women who have fallen victim to rape and other acts of violence because of unknowing smoking marijuana laced with who knows what. It happened to me, too. It happens often to women all over the country, often going unreported due to our own shame in misusing cannabis. Shattering the Stigma and educating ourselves on cannabis can provide us with a safe, natural alternative to remedy practically all of our health issues and can also give us the confidence to freely and joyfully consume cannabis, both medicinally and recreationally.

To say I've met some of the most incredible people from smoking cannabis would be an understatement. I've shared blunts with some of the most creative and revolutionary minds in our generation. Thinkers, musicians, artists, activists, teachers, poets, scholars, many hailing from places like Chicago, Los Angeles, Atlanta, Miami, New York, Maryland and Washington, D.C., all with one thing in common, our love and connection to the plant. In reclaiming cannabis as medicine, and using cannabis holistically, I've been able to support and connect with individuals, women and families in various cities and countries all over the world! I've been inspired. I am forever grateful.

These experiences are ultimately what led me to working as a junior gardener at a licensed medical cannabis cultivation center in Washington, D.C. in 2015. We were growing for mostly pediatric patients, elderly, hospice patients who were trying cannabis as a last resort, and were reporting great successes. It was an incredible time. Two months into cultivating cannabis, I found out that I was pregnant, and I was faced with a decisions that many expectant families have to make: the choice to consume cannabis during pregnancy. It is not an easy choice for most women, or their partners, in most cultures, in communities who don't have safe access, or where it is considered illegal. These women are ridden with fear and guilt about whether cannabis can hurt their babies or harm their pregnancy. This was not my reality.

I was knowledgeable about cannabis. I was working in the cannabis industry! Of course, I'd be supported in my decision, or so I thought.

Instead, I faced a lot of stigma, and discrimination, and resigned from my position after being demoted, underpaid, and disrespected in my position. It didn't matter how good I was with handling the grow rooms, or how easily and quickly I managed the hard labor of cultivation, I was pregnant. Five months pregnant, at that. I wanted to cower. I was embarrassed. Embarrassed to be pregnant, at a time when I was doing something that I truly loved and enjoyed doing. I felt like a quitter. Like I had been offered a chance at my living a dream, and I had it quickly snatched from me. I was ashamed, not of my own cannabis use or even the fact that I was pregnant—what consumed me was what everyone else may have been thinking or saying. While I was still growing cannabis, I was met with questions from family and friends like, "as long as you're not still smoking it, right…?" or "you not still smoking are you, g?"

When women like me, women who choose cannabis, announce that we are pregnant, rarely are we told congratulations. We're asked what we're going to do with it, or we're simply expected to abort it. No questions. The assumption and perception is that cannabis is bad during pregnancy. Says who? From my experience and the research I had done, cannabis was a safer alternative to many pharmaceutical drugs on the market currently offered to pregnant women. I had research to prove it. Even with research, and evidence-based information on cannabis use during pregnancy, the stigma persisted.

It was not my stigma alone. At around 8 months pregnant, I wobbled in to a community-based maternal health nonprofit in DC, where I had a job interview and was hired for the position of Intake Specialist. It was refreshing. I was enveloped in a village of Black women who were supporting other pregnant women. I was empowered. I was assigned a doula and given a bag of fresh food to take home. The very next day, I started conducting intake assessments for pregnant mothers, asking them questions about their pregnancy history and marijuana use, among other things. I was shocked by the many women who were using cannabis. I was not only shocked, I was happy to hear other women using cannabis as medicine to support nausea, vomiting, pain, depression and other issues during pregnancy, like me. I was pregnant, like them, and using cannabis, just as they were and at the same time I couldn't educate them on safely using cannabis, or even hint to them, or many of my co-workers, that I was also consuming it.

Like me, many of the women that I connected with during this time said that using cannabis use during pregnancy was instinctual. I started to wonder, just how many other women felt the same way. So I started my journey, connecting with other mothers who consumed cannabis. I started training as an independent doula, and received several certifications in cannabis education and holistic and herbal remedies. Traditionally, a doula is a birth professional and expert who provides mental, physical, and emotional support to women and families during pregnancy, childbirth, and postpartum, often providing natural herbal remedies and comfort measures to birthing families. I wanted to learn as much as I possibly could to support mothers, like me; Women and families who choose to consume cannabis, safely, traditionally, and holistically.

This is the journey of how I started to consume cannabis as an aid in healing past trauma related domestic violence, workplace violence, racism and white supremacy, post-traumatic slave syndrome and post-traumatic stress, depression and anxiety, turning the poison of my life experiences, into medicine to heal my body, my womb, and birth healthy, happy children and supporting other women and their families in doing the same.

The Cannabis Doula provides support for women and families who consume cannabis, especially during pregnancy, childbirth, and postpartum, by providing woman-centered cannabis education, holistic support, and cannabis caregiver services, in addition to holistic doula services and childbirth education.

Learn more at *www.thecannabisdoula.org*.

Disclaimer: Information contained within this book is for informational purposes only and is not intended to replace any medical advice or education. If you are considering consuming cannabis during pregnancy, or while nursing, please consult with your primary care provider and a qualified cannabis practitioner.

Like Water
For Chocolate City

for july fourth

I experience racism everyday.
maybe I always have
and was just blind to it
in Chicago.

maybe the DMV is just
one of those places
or damn.
maybe I attract it.

Recently the things I see
and experience
on a daily basis,
to and from work
out and about,
is shocking.
degrading.
crushing even.

Though my heart
becomes stronger,
my mind
and my tongue
a bit more sharp,
sometimes I even have to look around to see
if anyone has *seen what I just seen,*
saw what just happened, or
even if *somebody was gone say something.*
but maybe I'm tripping.

or worse,
maybe as a society we have become
so accustomed to our own filth,
that which they call racism and prejudice
but never say out loud.
maybe amerikkka.

so comfortable in shit and consumed in it
ingrained.
so deeply rooted
in hate,
that we can't even smell it
anymore.

Racism comes up with the sun
but does not sleep at night.
It's hot and humid.
and I can't breathe.

It's gentrification.
and I want to see my people.

G.O.A.T

When people ask me where I'm from
I tell them.
I don't try to talk proper or speak their lingo.
I use my own slang.
ain't is still my favorite word. and finna.
G goes before and after.
I don't wear what they wear,
we don't walk the same,
and I ain't finna assimilate.
If we do in fact like the same music,
mine is always better.

"Chicago."
Head up, proud, boastful.
"Oh, damn," they say
It's always an oh, the pitiful kind of *oh*.
"That's a cool city...
but I hear its rough out there..."
It's always a *but*.
"So which part you from?"

"South Side."

"Damn, that's fucked up,
that's like the worse place to be from."

I cock my head slowly
toward my right shoulder
brows lowered
eyes squinted
and I wonder

how anyone
can speak so demeaningly
and so matter-of-factly
about a person's

home.

where I was born.
where I breathed
life.
where I laughed,
cried,
played, learned
and struggled.
for

23 years.

flame up

Moments like this seem long overdue,
like a clouded heart
or a lazy spirit
waiting to be released.

Strong scents of incense
carrying the voice of erykah badu,
like how candles fill a room
and let down your guard,
you fill my soul
and I explode.

Between the blaze of your mouth
and the daze of my eyes.
High.
We float.

Soul mates at any rate
We ain't got no other friends.
I admired you
and broke you
up all at once.
Caressing every bit of you
with the tips of my fingers,
to make you as strong
as the last time.

On the line
between love and addiction,
rolled up tightly
with the lust of my warm tongue,
as wet as always.
I'll be patient
though my need is dire,
taking pieces of my soul
and lighting it on fire.

Deep inhales that set sail
the feel of euphoria
and timeless ecstasy
exhaling the angst of lost desire.
The passion comes quickly
when you're
lit
on fire
and hot
between my lips.

the coming home to

I give the boys something to hope for,
like the coming home to.
I give them a place to love
and a space to share
I give them the care that was not honored
by their mothers
and dismissed by their fathers.
I give them kisses.
and touch them in
places remiss by past lovers

I give them the confidence to build kingdoms
and the wisdom to plant trees.
I give them the strength of a hundred men
armored in esteem and harmony.
Benevolence.
The Black Man,
praised highly and exalted.
I give them the knowledge that confirms it.

I give them the melanin in me,
the yellow of the sun,
and the blue of the sea.
I give them
truth.
and share my energy.
They ignore the leaves so
I teach them their roots.

I am the muse
behind their artwork
and the words behind their inquires.
I am the Queen
yet,
they give me
nothing.

full moon

I dance under the moon
in celebration of what's to come
feet planted firmly in soil
embracing every blade of grass
every branch. even the
rocks that seek to stub my
toe. hands fully outstretched
reaching for the sky
hugging the stars in praise and satisfaction
with nighttime. it's peaceful
solitude. it's honesty
the imagination that
comes with night
sparks the most
profound
and sweet
creativity that one
can only hope will
last til morning
will last during the day--
when our childhood selves
are not welcomed to play--
our desire suppressed
with everyday realisms
how brutal
a world
but then
how beautiful.
the glory that comes
with the setting of the sun.
I dance under the moon
and I create life.

like water for chocolate city

Between the cracks of government buildings
leaks the tears of Africans.
A city once flowing,
like the river, basking in the sweetness of la chocolat
Now dank with disorder and confusion.
Corruption resides where love once was.
Violence and drugs polluted,
brainwashed
a Black people
leaving history diluted
the anger of gentrification refuted,
stunting growth
for generations to come.

Respect undone
and replaced with hate.
An invisible enemy
welcomed brutality and sin.
Oppression
is strong in Babylon.

Blood drips from the leaves.
trees begging
to return to freedom.
One man's free world
is but a prison for those who built it,
for those of whom lie buried beneath it.

Between the dark shadows of government buildings
looms dark faces
of homelessness and poverty.
mis-educating the very Negroes
who descended here
baring the fruit of shame,
a slave by any other name
is still

a slave.

Slaves
in the farmlands
of Zimbabwe,
Slaves in US jails and
slaves in our school hallways
Slaves to corporate greed
Slaves in the streets of DC,
from Baltimore to LA
& everywhere in between.

They've enslaved a whole people
to profit from a crop
Cash from hemp and cotton
Lashes from whips
Chains and ships
People thrown overboard
And forgotten.

They enslaved a whole people
to profit from a crop.
Cash from hemp and cotton.
Outlawed the plants
and the seeds
that healed
the bodies of many.
Poisoned the food and flower,
the water
in Chocolate City.

Weed, to us, is medicine.
They've polluted it like water
in cities like Flint.
Cannabis cures, heals everything
for them, a place to profit.

There is no healing trauma
for Black families causing
disease and illness

to prosper.

Cannabis aligns
our chakras.
Bringing balance & peace,
Joining yin and yang.
Giving birth to Black
Enlightenment.

Grams said
government-sponsored
abortions
are akin to eugenics.
Misinformation,
and racism has
populated our politics.
Propaganda fed to women
since the very beginning,
so that we forget.

They've colonized the herbs,
outlawed the midwives,
calling Grams a witch.
It's the job of white insecurity
is to disguise Black worth.
Leaving no images
of Black women
reflected in the river.
Black mothers
left dying to birth.

Black children diagnosed
with diseases,
born to a people
working minimum wage,
corporate slaves
in neighborhoods,
ravaged
and torn to pieces.
No clean water

for Chocolate City.

Slave labor has never stopped,
while opioid use increases.
Slaves to every industry,
in every town,
What happened
to Chocolate City?

Reparations are due
From all of you
Making money from our blood
Flowing,
Flowing in the streets
Our ancestors
Speak
through us.

The water
will continue to rise
and The Fire Next Time
will be higher
and higher.

Until the prison
gates open,
and the broken
are no longer
tired.

Until Black mothers
labor without any pain
and our medicinal plants
are free.

Cannabis cures
Heals everything
Like Water
for Chocolate City.

the queen bee

don't call me no B.
don't run when you see me
waving your hands and arms
ridiculously.

don't kill me
with your eyes.
forcing me to fall victim to your
stereotypes and perceived notions.

don't call me no B.
don't criminalize Blackness.
don't marginalize Brown skin.
don't kill Black men...
womb-men
or children.

Everyone hates bees.
but if the Bees were to disappear
from the surface of the earth,
man would have no more
than four years to live.

B is for Black.
and unapologetically so
Black is power.
Black Power.
Black was the first color used in art.
Art imitates life.

If the universe was Black
before God created light
God is Black.
Black is The Standard.
my melanin out stands
any disease,

dis-ease
we
are the seeds
of our ancestors.
They harvest in our skin.
Kin.
The Creators of Life.
The Asiatic Black Man.

I may act like a bitch sometimes.
but don't call me no B.
because
"Ain't I a Woman?
I have ploughed
and planted
and gathered into barns,
and no man
can head me."

So don't call me no B.

"If the first woman
God ever made
was strong enough to turn
the world upside down
all alone,
these women together
ought to be able to turn it back,
and get it right side up again."

Leaving the B-word with something better.
Be the boldness basking
in the beauty that beholds that
B-word.

I am Pro-Her.
Pro-Sojourner Truth, *"Ain't I a Woman?"*
Pro-Maya Angelou, *"I Know Why the Caged Birds Sings."*
Pro-Little Black girl from 79th Street
and I don't play that Bitch word.

so don't call me no B
because my Blackness bothers you.

I will pollinate
every sunflower
every tree
sustaining animals
providing the necessary
essentials for human life.
you can not kill me.
or the honey bee!
The Queen Bee.
I will not be moved.

the personification of the universe

"Like an artist with no art form
she became dangerous."
I was treacherous in my lust
and a menace to unrequited passion.
Not caught up in the rapture of love,
but rather
the irony of making love
and having sex.

I apologize.

I am art.
Like Nola Darling
And Nina Mosley
I'd paint men in primary colors.
Indigo.

I'd write poems of romantic tragedies
describing old lovers.
Drawing shapes to take space
and reflect time.
Complete symphonies
harmonizing
the melody of beating hearts.
Images capturing a scene
a perfect as God's eye.

I no longer settle for the idea
that man was born to die
He is alive to create.

Everything else
is dangerous.

our father

To the men
whose hearts were crushed
by their mothers long before
we had the pleasure
of being their lovers.
To the men
whose fathers left them
and hurt them
more deeply than
they could ever hurt us.

To the men who thought
that our bodies
and our hearts
were mutually exclusive,
refusing to take one with the other.

For our father who forgot
to teach us
that having sex
wasn't the same
as saying thank you.

To the men who could never
just say *i love you* back.
for our father who never told us,
and our mother who didn't show us,
that we were pretty
and that no make up
could ever produce art
comparable to what God painted.

If love is what the Moon
looks to the Sun for,
this is to the men
who could never

see us as an entity,
who never understood
that complimenting
a part of me
meant loving themselves entirely.

For our father
who never knew
that our time with him
should have been
our first real date.
To the men who turned
into fake-homies,
ex-lovers,
and old friends
without our permission.

For our father who
didn't teach us
that saying no
in our heads
meant just the same
as saying it aloud.

To the men who never thought
to make back up our beds.
For our father who
never saw himself
as our first male friend.
To the men who never wanted us
for being too lonely,
and for our father
who couldn't bare the thought
of being alone
so much
that he stayed away.

To the men
who didn't want us
because we were always fighting

for something—
probably for our father,
who made us weak
by teaching us
and showing us
that women can't fight.

To the men
who wouldn't fix
what was broken,
For our father,
(and probably our mother)
who broke us.

This is to the men
whose hearts were
crushed by their mothers
long before we had the pleasure
of being their lovers.
To the men whose fathers
left them and hurt them
more deeply than they could ever hurt us.

I wrote this
and I cried for you,
and not because you made me
or because I needed to,
but because *you* did.
so I released it, and
I cried for you.

thank you
for associating me
with your perception
of what love is.
I got love for you, too.

evolution of the Black man
in amerikkka

blood in the sea
blood on the leaves
blood in the soil
blood in the streets.

another dark figure
outlined between
yellow traffic paint.

we are not niggers.

Our blood stains
the white man's uniform
crucifying us.
Denying us
the right to breathe
the right to be free.
Teaching us to pray to a white God,
for a white Christmas,
a big house with white picket fences.
white-washing our existence.

It is not okay for you to cross here.
Candles and stuffed bears
surrounding crosses,
balloons, cards made from school children
for hurt moms with desolate wombs,
for desolate moms
with hurt wombs,
left picking up the pieces.

Exposing the Black skeletons
in amerikkka's closet,
condescendingly mourning our losses
by insisting on non-violent marches.

Hands up, Don't shoot!
and every time they do
roses line the street to conceal
the blood stained concrete.

We been thinking
maybe that they grew there.
That the blood somehow
planted seeds to uproot
springing forth the revolution,
once again.
you will see us.

The Evolution of
The Black Man.
These Black boys
been Jesus.

Now,
is the resurrection.

**you can never love someone
as much as you can miss them.**

I'm forcing these words
across paper here because
I can't bear to hear
your voice anymore.

My fingers have a hard time
dialing your phone number
and I wonder if you even miss me
at all.

I am afraid
that I forgot what you
look like.

I've avoided mirrors
so that I won't see you.
I'm starting to wonder
where I came from,
or better yet, whom.

The scent of your perfume
on my sweater left months ago.
I can no longer fit your old clothes.
I have nothing
but throwback Thursdays
and flashback Fridays
to look forward to.
A shallow past.

How easy it is
for you to run away
I guess you taught me that.

I want to know
where your soul

has been hiding
and what demons
killed your spirit,
shielding hate in your heart.
Or is it your Self
that you can't live with?

I am terrified that
you are the woman
I am trying not to be.
Bitter about love,
cynical, and unhappy.

"Never put all your
eggs in one basket," you said,
and yet you placed four
of your eggs in one
and lost yourself
in passing.

I question whether
you ever loved yourself,
whether the scars
and the bruises
on your skin
has left you permanently
damaged, broken, by men.

You ain't never love me right.
Your hug never felt as tight
as it was supposed to.
Perhaps you're too weak
to understand karma and too lost
to demand faith.

The cause of self-hate
is the effect of loneliness.
The whole universe
would explode,
my whole heart

would be empty,
the breath in my lungs
would become so scarce
the strongest wind couldn't
fill them up again.
Breathless,
because I need you.
not flowers
smoked to hide
eyes that look like yours.

I exhale,
and live,
in every
memory of you.

I will not settle for the idea
that missing you,
you not being here,
is greater than
your love.

war

Words trapped in the back
of my throat
unspoken.

Half-broken hearts
waiting to be found out.
Lost against the softness of morning,
My, how night escapes us.

Hoping that the light of the sun
will illuminate the shadows of past lovers—
I am leaving them.
Forgotten at the sight of you.
Love, in likeness, made whole through your touch.

My mind eases at the sound of your voice.
I want to love you so bad.
I want to trade sleepless nights
engulfed in loneliness and angst
For 3am conversations of building a nation
Waiting all day just to do it again.
To spend hours entwined in each other's dreams

I want to give the stillness
of quiet walls echoing mere uncertainty
For the richness of your laughter,
And the pleasure of your adornment.
I want to expose myself to you.
Stripped down to the core of my identity.
Unmasked.
Unclothed of past abandonment.

Left longing for attachment,
Wrapped in sin,
Lusting for anything that will have me.
My eyes have not seen love.

My body has never been touched by it.
My tongue has yet to recognize
the taste of love on the skin of any man.

If loving is leaving,
then that's all I know how to do.
Abused.
Battered with repeat offenses
of broken promises
never to be made whole anyway,
or recognized as truth.

Disguising the infatuation
of a one night stand
left fallen and loose
with the inflictions
from redressing old wounds.
partly given by bruised men
holding no intention of
seeing me through til morning

When everything is made new and the
lies of last night are left open to view:
A place where sex and loyalty
have no commitment to one another.
we were never friends,
how can we be lovers?

We are at war but fighting for nothing.
Only left to grapple with the reality
That we will never be together
We will never be free.
Centuries of tattered families
leave no room for me.

The womb of Black women,
once baring kings
now produces genetically
modified black youth.
Building foundations

upon white lies
for an illusion of home.
Poorly grown
and crumbling under pressure.

We are at war
but fighting for nothing.

We are at war but fighting for nothing.

do the whole world a favor

Come
do the whole world a favor.
quiet my roaring heart
with your love.
soothe my soul at two a.m.
take one for the team.

catch me.
tie me down.
build me up.
impregnate me with you knowledge,
my God.

come, do the whole world a favor.
and love.
create with me.
Let us manifest a world
as beautiful and as powerful
as the coming together of our spirits.

Your queen and my king
embodying new realities
and complete truths
tip the scales of justice
in favor of just us.

Let us build pyramids
and configure mathematical theories
to express our love.

Watch the stars align for you
and the sun pay homage
to the moon.
Leaving sculptures of our adoration
all over the world,
let me be art to you.

Plant trees in me,
deeply rooted.
let us rewrite history
by watering seeds.
Produce a rich harvest in me.

For we are alchemy.
Let us turn this lead to gold.
Let us go love supreme.
Come.
Come do the whole
world a favor
with your love
move me.
turn me right side up.

black girl blue

"Ain't no sunshine when she's gone
It's not warm when she's away.
Ain't no sunshine when she's gone
And she's always gone too long
Anytime she goes away.
Anytime she goes away..."

Scars like thin slits
fill the spaces
of her wrist to her forearm
like the stripes of a tiger's back.
carved out of self-hate and confusion.
the illusion of love is always deceit.
my mind often flashes back to images of her.
The innocence of childhood
is too often overcome with darkness.
Generations of despair
inherited at adolescence
like a Rites of Passage.

Insecurity passed down
from mother to daughter.
I once asked what made you do it,
slit your wrists as you do,
but inside I already knew.
"Physical pain distracts
from the emotional wounds."
you told me,
then showed me
how to rest in peace.
The pain of being a
Black girl,
blue.

"Ain't no sunshine when she's gone
Only darkness every day.

48

Ain't no sunshine when she's gone
And this house just ain't no home
Anytime she goes away."

Purple bruises are not flattering
on Black skin,
especially women.
neither are black eyes
or swollen lips gifts
to be worn with pride.
So she'd hide under
expensive clothes to mask
how cheap he made her feel.
My mom looked good in all black,
stunning,
as she mourned the death of my father's soul
each time he'd hit her.
we all moved a little closer to hell
as they rumbled at its doorstep.

I once wondered
how you could awaken
everyday as you do.
Left battered and empty
to cook breakfast for a man
who abused you.
But inside I already knew.
physical pain distracts
from the emotional wounds
The pain of being a
Black girl,
blue.

"Ain't no sunshine when she's gone
Only darkness every day.
Ain't no sunshine when she's gone
And this house just ain't no home
Anytime she goes away."

I'll never really know

what happened to you.
What agony you had to bare
to inherit your stripes.
I'll never understand
all you had to go through.
what trauma must now engulf you.
We want too badly
to be like our mothers.
the pain of being a
Black girl, blue.

I stand on the shoulders
of giants. warriors, Black women, queens
often defeated but never wavering.
We will not be moved.
"pick up your crown,
live in your glory until we are all free,"
they told me,
"Feel everything so deeply,
so immensely that the world will move
for you."

I am a product of their victory
and the shadow of their triumph.
I am, because we are.
here is faith
here is hope
And here is love.
these three
but the greatest of these,
is you.

for all Black girls, blue.

"Ain't no sunshine when she's gone
Only darkness every day.
Ain't no sunshine when she's gone
And this house just ain't no home
Anytime she goes away."

doomed for her demise

Free Zimbabwe
Under the crown
King Mugabe

Free us of
Capitalistic tyranny
Globally oppressing collectivity,
to unveil individual corruption and greed—
power or need?
Seeds grown by black farmers
to build white supremacy.

Sanctions placed
like a noose
upon the neck
of the most productive Black nation
to feed the white faces of amerikkkan corporations,
Black labor to favor their politics, tricks,
families suffer as time tics,
whole communities strangling, gasping from its grip.
Black economics stripped
and crumbling away.

There are new slaves
in the farmlands of Zimbabwe.
All hail king Mugabe.
I'm restoring the equilibrium
to liberate—
introducing free minds to strategy
it is time disintegrate
the very system that they use:

Who controls the mass distribution of the purest produce?
Who grows all the food and dies from not eating?
Who widens the gap of wealth distribution?
Who dies from disease spread by western institutions?

Who creates lies to hinder political solutions?
The same people who infiltrate the peace, and brainwash the youth.
The same people who instill fear,
fill the air with pollutants &
mass media produced illusion.

They've contaminated the water
and privatized the sea.
The same people
who haze human beings
and praise technology.
The same people
who block trade and place embargoes,
sponsor Islamic Terrorist Activity
and torture at Guantanamo Bay.

They build relations out of hate
to impose infractions.
They mention God
to guise their evil actions.
Resulting in imperialism and poverty.
They've murdered millions
and called it democracy.

An anomaly to us
is just business to them.
Disgracing our motherland,
spreading world wide corruption.
And famine.
Amerikkka and all her horror,
disrupting harmony and community
across the diaspora.

Redistribute the wealth.
Health and eduction
are not luxuries only
afforded to the rich,
Our families stripped by U.S. indignations
the most inhumane nation,
the United States of Tyranny.

Unfair and unholy territory.

Pedagogy of hate
as humankind awaits her fate
Pedagogy of hate
as humankind awaits her fate.
Pedagogy of hate
as humankind awaits her fate.

She is doomed
for her demise.

education

Tainted images of what Black is,
that is the world we live in.
Unconsciously hating our skin as if
Africa didn't make us beautiful enough.

Where every system fails us unjustly,
the ugly reality of broken families.
A broke people, weakened
but we pledge allegiance.
I hate that shit.

Tainted images of what Black is
back then we were hanged from trees
to teach us our roots.
89,790 days of enslavement
and hell-bent on disguising the truth,
forgetting to include the profound Blackness
in which light itself was created.

Life weighted on the shoulders of Black men
back when one of us was 3/5ths of one of them.
Corruption in the minds of Black youth
I don't remember learning about Fred Hampton in school...
or the African Burial Grounds in NYC.
We built an entire nation *(again)* and it wasn't until 1993
that they considered it "history."

If the department of defense
was built on the land of former slave descendants
then who's free lives are they defending?
Freedman's Village sounds a lot like my neighborhood,
Englewood, and Auburn Gresham.
We're the descendants of the same people
constantly unconsciously uprooted.
Like crack was polluted
through us back in the day.

they are the ones giving our
little boys these guns.
I can keep going but I'm hoping the war ends
this fucked up system.
They make us hate us
so that we will kill each other
then blame violence
on the lack of education.

there goes spring

I do not like winter.
Not December through early March
Not during the darkest hour
of my moon,
when the tears stream from unknown
and abandoned places.
Not the faces I see in the mirror
of greyness and gloom,
a person longing for real,
real freedom, and life, and love.

I do not like winter.
I do not like what quiet sounds
like after 10pm.
I don't like the
smell of an empty room.

But then, at the flicker of
a candle, like the
smell of cotton.
There goes spring.

r.i.p.
Mitchell

black girls like us

Queens.
Flaunting like so.
Learning to love every curl and kink
on our yet acquainted heads.
Behold,
your crown.
Our kingdom.
Shea, Coconut, Jojoba is Just for Me
Afro picks and afro pics
in place of where perms used to be.

Maybe someone should have told us,
they won't know how to love your hair,
Black girls like us.
Queens.
Unknowingly so.
Learning to love men who don't love themselves
Hoping to find the warmth of our hearts in their beds
Familiar feelings with unfamiliar men,
Maybe our daddies should have told us
They won't know how to love you,
Black girls like us.
Queens.
Rightfully so.
Bold, intelligent, beautiful
Our bodies like art,
as intricate as our mind.
Eyes like Horus.
Duafe.

Maybe I should have told you —
they won't know what to do with, to, or for
Black girls like us, who
go back
and we fetch it.

1511 franklin

I longed for you
and not in a way that most lovers
would normally do.

my mind wanted
to live within yours
even offering to pay rent there
with hopes of finding a home sturdy enough
to hold every thing she held
packed away in suitcases
and open enough for the sun
to flow through freely.

a place so fruitful and nurturing
that flowers could even grow there,
so lovely that the rain
would feel invited to fall on us
just so that it'll never know what it's like to leave the sky
making us forget
that we were ever getting wet in the first place.

My hands wanted to feel you.
From the coconut oil braised curls
on the nape of your neck
to the soft brown buttery skin
that you never imagined
could be touched so sincerely.

My legs were ready to devote themselves to you.
Ready to take on every
command that was placed upon them,
passionately wrapping themselves around you
and not releasing
until they understood what it really felt like
to want
someone.

The way your body
filled parts of my being,
places that I never knew existed, now had feeling.
My heart
seeing what she, herself,
had been missing,
the way you'd stay for hours at her whim,
your words slowing stitching up every
scrape and scar that had even been forced upon her.
You were even offering to
hold on to pieces
of my thoughts for me
so that I wouldn't get too tired
of baring the pain
that man and womb-man
should be sharing.

Then showering
me with long kisses
and passionate stares,
how dare you make me weak.
and think.
I will speak circles around you.
giving your name
all of the power
that I could muster
and lust for.

Soft caresses
of beautiful Black skin
hidden between covers--
just so that the walls
wouldn't get jealous
because I longed for you.
and no longer for their silence.
The peacefulness of what they've shown me
of what it's like being alone
but not lonely.
not searching for a strong hand
and loving eye to care for me.

and when I found that in you,
I wondered
was it really you that I longed for.
or the idea that
something so gentle
So pure
and peaceful
can exist
beyond
my walls.

trayvon martin

Throwback to when hoodies
were up for
Trayvon Martin.
To when we
were protesting,
rallying,
signing petitions
just to get Zimmerman to trial.
Then he was acquitted.
That moment changed me.
That year.
From the time Trayvon Martin
was killed to the moment
they announced
the acquittal of George Zimmerman.
Things shifted.
What was so unbelievable to us
then is happening everyday now.
and my hoodie is still up.
But this time,
fast forward to today,
I am no longer
 waiting for justice
to be served,
but rather,
I am
taking it.

Happy Birthday,
Trayvon Martin.

i love you. see you soon. take care.

She's addicted to leaving.
It's the only time she hears
I love you.

The only time she experiences
love
in an outward,
physical
expression.

She doesn't love herself.
She doesn't know how,
so she comes,
and goes.

For an *I love you*
and a *be safe.*
I'll see you soon.

Waiting.

for someone
to beg her
to stay.

She hopes
and dreams,
But she always leaves.

Until next time,
iloveyouseeyousoontakecare.

ode to dr. maya angelou

I called you my favorite poet
In 5th grade,
maybe before
still in ball knockers
and barrettes.
I recited your poetry verbatim, or
as though I'd imagine you'd say them.

Ten years old,
maybe eleven—
reciting Still I Rise
and watching Poetic Justice
talking about diamonds
at the meeting of my thighs!

Does it come as a surprise that your words
spoke power into me?
I studied you, intently.
As boys did superman or batman,
or anybody doing superhero things
saving the world sparking their wildest dreams.
Heroes to them,
as you were to me,
I called you
my favorite poet.

I danced for you, you know,
On 78th and Throop
where hundreds of us gathered and we sat at your feet.
I remember like
it was yesterday,
you stood from your seat
Unable to stand alone, you cried,
gracefully,
humbling tears
you bowed

to me.

When I first understood what it meant
to be a Black woman
in America,
I called you my favorite poet.
your words wrapped around me tighter
than my mother's embrace, warm and sweet,
when no hugs were afforded
to Black girls
who dared to dream—
but were not given any heroes.
you were that to me.

grabbing the world
by the lapels
and freeing my own caged birds
it was my day of birth
the day you died.
I paid homage to you
that night,
Dr. Angelou,
at Bus Boys with the poets.
Reading your words
to Madiba,
His Day is Done,
thinking who would write such words
for you when your day too,
is done.
who would write
the greatest poem,
for the greatest
poet known?

I called you my favorite poet,
Marguerite Ann Johnson,
Dr. Maya Angelou.
May we grieve
for the voice of
Black womanhood

of which you
phenomenally
declared
we wear our crowns,
and dance.

I grieve for little Black girls
who may never know you
existed who may have never
felt you
and cried
for your words.

I mourn for little Black girls who printed
lines of your work
on their bedroom walls
or secretly in their journals.
Because even in your silence,
you gave us hope.

I've come to learn
that Black girls don't talk sometime.
and that writing is a powerful weapon.
and that even when no one wants to hear what should be said,
we need to speak truth anyway.

I too have a song to sing.
I too sing of freedom.
I too, a caged bird

freed.

dear love

you know why
I'm not mad at you?
because I bleed for you.
and for every other intelligent
and beautiful Black man just like you—
who can't possibly imagine how anyone could love them.
or what that even feels like.
how thoroughly brainwashed
you have been
to hate yourselves
that you can't even
love you
let alone allow me
to love you too.
there is no revolution without love.
there is no fight worth fighting
nor life worth living.
no art will ever
be as beautiful.
I wonder what
rendered you incapable of love.
what has taken your heart from your chest
and replaced it with despair?
I wonder what
my loneliness
would look like
on a Black man.
Does it creep up in the middle
of the night making dreams impossible?
Does it make you choke?
wrapping it's cold white fingers around your neck until
you call out
for a god that doesn't
even look like you.

Do you have peace of mind?

or are your thoughts
louder than your own voice. have you realized
that no one can hear you,
if your heart
doesn't speak
first.

I wonder what my hurt would look like
on a Black man.
do you even know what a real hug
is should to feel like?
the way you collapse
into my arms,
I wondered if you had
ever been touched before.

How do you survive in a world
that is taught to hate you?
Can you even stand to look in the mirror?
I am sorry that you were a criminal before you were a boy,
then a monster, much less than a man.
I'm sorry, I should have noticed.
I should have reminded you
that by looking in the mirror,
you would see all of humanity
in your flesh and the power of the world
in your eyes.
I should have warned you,
that they'd never see you as an equal,
because you are superior.
that they'd never treat you as a man
because you are a God

and a King
amongst
His people.

Dear love,
until you learn to love,
I will always love you.

gemini

self-fulfilling prophecies
that were forced upon me
true beliefs of lost histories
waiting for the moment
to say I love you.
long stares that fill in the blanks
of missing words
short breaths and unsteady heartbeats
weeks, months, years even yearn
for the sweetness of your time
the smooth outline of blackness
private romance shared
between two lovers
lusting to be together,
searching for one another.
love nowhere to be found.
not a sunflower.
not a piece of chocolate
melting between fingers.
no music playing between kisses.
just wishes and thoughts
of unpursued passions.
dreams of loving you,
loving dreams of you,
love dreams of you
whoever
you are.

he said I couldn't

Old habits die hard
So I'm taking a piece from Eve's Book.
Picking fruit from the wrong tree
I'm lonely and he just likes the way it looks.
He's lovely and loves me
But can't,
so he won't.
As if his mind had the power
To tell his heart what to do
and choose too.
Something forbidden is
Always ridden in taboo.

He said I couldn't,
written off with no regard
like the apple
wasn't bitten.
I wished he
wouldn't have
thrown feelings
I wasn't supposed to catch.
Sharing a heart
that won't attach
with no intent
to fall through
I said "I love you..."
And he said I couldn't,
because she does...
I don't know if
I was making him love me
or begging him to.
The misery of eating
this fruit I call you.

who is like God?

Consuming
thoughts of consummating ideas.
I finally know what love is.
It is two hearts that dream
of the same revolution.
At the same time.
In the same language.
And hands that sing of romance.
It is dancing eyes
and hopeful lips.
It is when the mind makes sense
of the heart's purpose.

It just feels,
"Good,"
He said.

Revolutionary Motherhood

War on the Wombs of Black Women
December 24, 2014

As a Black woman and feminist, it propels me to make certain connections between my Blackness and my womanhood. I often find it necessary to step outside of myself to examine both spheres that are equally oppressed alone and even more so when combined. To be Black and to be a woman is to live as two oppressed minorities in one.

It is to be expected that as a woman, I will be deemed less than my male counterparts, not deserving of equal pay, and not valued for my education or my opinion. I am eye-candy; only good for my looks, performance in the bedroom and in the kitchen, and relatively nothing else. As a woman in America, that comes with the territory. As a Black woman though, it is expected of me to be sexually exploitative and deviant. To be loud and reckless. White women often look and speak to us belittlingly like we are little girls, much less women, and white men seek us to fulfill their often erotic desires and sexual fantasies. There is money to be made in the exploitation of Black women and girls. From our hair and nails, supplied to us by billion-dollar industries not owned by us, to our bodies being sold on corners or through underground sex industries by Black men and white men alike. Our asses being mere advertisements in mainstream music videos. Where did this anti-Black woman culture come from?

Where everything else did–slave culture. During slavery, especially after the Trans-Atlantic Slave Trade was halted, white slave masters would set up slave farms for the breeding of Black women to make more slaves. They would gather Black women, some as young as 12, putting a male slave in charge to perform provocative dances so that the slave-master could have his pick of the best, most attractive slave to rape and impregnate. Enslaved Black men would also be forced to mate with the women and girls. Slave masters would force slaves to perform orgies while they watched and participated. Often as incentive, Black women would be granted freedom or special treatment if they bore a certain number of children into slavery, 15 or more.

In a series of slave narratives, women would speak on the jealousy and abuse that they'd experience from the slave masters' wives. The sex practices during slavery, I found, are rarely spoken of because the practices were so obscene and the ramifications on bodies of Black women still exist today.

The war on the wombs of Black women have always been in place. By war on the womb, I am talking about the abuse and neglect of Black women's bodies especially in relation to bearing and raising healthy children into adulthood. *Any injustice against black children is a facet in the war on the wombs of Black women.* The murder of Black youth (like Trayvon Martin, Mike Brown, Aiyana Jones, Tamir Rice, Antonio Martin, etc. etc.) by police or vigilantes is an attack on Black women more than anything. It is a message being sent that any product of our wombs is not worthy of life. The mass media messages and music that praise and uphold violent lifestyles influences our children to hate themselves, to hate us, and to kill each other and themselves. Black women are subjected to disease through chemically induced food and water in urban areas which contributes to many types of illnesses that affect the womb can cause damage for generations.

A fact-sheet by the Center for American Progress on the State of Black Women in America, reported the health disparities in African American women:

- One in four African American women are uninsured. This lack of health insurance, along with other socioeconomic factors, continues to contribute to the dire health issues African American women face.
- Hypertension is more prevalent among African American women than any other group of women: 46 percent of African American women 20 years of age and older have hypertension, whereas only 31 percent of white women and 29 percent of Hispanic women in the same age bracket do.
- While white women are more likely to have breast cancer, African American women have higher overall mortality rates from breast cancer. Every year, 1,722 African American women die from breast cancer—an average of five African American women per day. Chlamydia and gonorrhea infection rates for African American women are 19 times higher than those of white women.
- African American women have higher rates of human papillomavirus, or HPV, and cervical cancer, with mortality rates double those of white women.

74

- African American women represent 65 percent of new AIDS diagnoses among women.
- African American women experience unintended pregnancies at three times the rate of white women.
- Black women are four times more likely to die from pregnancy-related causes, such as embolism and pregnancy-related hypertension, than any other racial group.
- Birth rates for teenage African American women from ages 15 to 19 decreased by 7 percent from 2011 to 2012.
- African American women have the highest rates of premature births and are more likely to have infants with low or very low birth weights.
- African American infants are more than 2.4 times more likely as white infants to die in their first year of life.
- Only 35 percent of African American lesbian and bisexual women have had a mammogram in the past two years, compared to 60 percent of white lesbian and bisexual women.

I present all of this because we, as Black women, should know where we stand, as to make conscious decisions for the sake of ourselves and generations to come. Not only do we have to fight for each other against the oppressive forces of patriarchy that seeks to exploit our bodies but we must continue to be on the front lines in working against police brutality, white supremacy, and the psychological trauma that our children constantly fall victim to. How can we do this?

The National Center of Education Statistics as reported by the U.S. Census found that Black women are the highest group by race and gender to be enrolled in colleges and universities. We must use our education to benefit the Black community, only. We must continue to establish our own businesses and not work for anyone but ourselves. We have to speak up. Even at the expense of being labeled the "Angry Black Bitch," we have to speak our truths.

We have to speak against men who exploit us as women and corporations and systems that exploit Black labor and Black culture. More than anything, we have to heal our wombs. We have been subjected to torture for generations before us, and for many of us, in our own lifetimes as well. We have to get in tune with the universe by eating natural foods and healing ourselves naturally and holistically.

We have to love ourselves and teach our youth how to love themselves. We have to love our men, even when they are not deserving. We have to teach them to be Kings, to love themselves, and we have to teach them how to treat us as Queens, rightfully so.

Successfully fighting this war on the wombs of Black women involves us becoming conscious to all efforts brought forth by society to devalue and erase us. We must educate ourselves and train ourselves to be wiser and faster. We have to reprogram and teach our own children. We have to heal our wombs. Our wombs gave birth to an entire universe, all of mankind was nursed by us. We have the power. We have to use it.

For more information on what I've referenced, research:
- Slave farms, slave breeding, sex practices during slavery.
- Download the State of Black Women in America report and share with family and friends.
- Have a discussion and learn your family medical history.
- Stop the cycle.

For womb work and spiritual healing:
- Check out Queen Afua's Sacred Woman for ancient kemetic rituals and womb wellness.
- Join a womb healing circle.
- Incorporate yoni steaming into your wellness routine
- Build.

one

I was thinking a lot about marijuana and I really became interested in learning about the different types of cannabis plants and strains. I decided to start my quest for knowledge through google. First, I wanted to know the most common types of weed largely because I was trying to find out what type of weed I had been smoking. I searched around for the difference between "loud" and "mid" because those were the terms I heard most often, and probably have most often smoked—though I still don't know the actual names, just their level of highness. I then go to YouTube to search for videos on marijuana, specifically factual based information, like documentaries that you won't find anywhere else. I wanted the real shit. I really feel like there is so much more to marijuana than the government would like the public to know in order to profit the large companies that fuel the economy.

I learned about how there was some type of ban placed on marijuana growth and use by the U.S. government during the Nixon administration, I believe, so that people would turn to companies for things like medicine and prescription pills to treat things that have been proven to be treatable or manageable by marijuana use (i.e. cancer, depression, nausea, headaches, the list goes on for mental illnesses that can also be managed by marijuana use) and proper stimulation of the Endocannabanoid System. Which I learned is throughout our entire bodies and helps to regulate the same things that cannabis (marijuana) manages.

Get it? Cannabis= Endocannabinoid System

There is an obvious link there. The research suggested that by smoking or using marijuana and allowing cannabis to interact with the Endocannabinoid System the plant actually stimulates the productivity of the system.
Regulates hunger: therefore lowering the income in food sales, weight loss industry, etc. *Treats illnesses and reduces likelihood of others*: lowering the annual income in medicine, health care, etc.
Building an economy off of a plant (nature) vs. building off of companies and industries (nurture)

Research therapeutic practices used with marijuana.

Better In Tune With The Infinite
Written for Black Girl In Om | May 12, 2015

When we find ourselves on the cusp of reaching our dreams, nearly overcome by the fatigue of late nights and the hunger of much deserved success and acknowledgment it is easy to lose sight of our true selves. One's personal journey is never easy, in actuality; following our dreams with all that we have is probably the hardest thing that we will ever undertake. We are tested every step of the way so that when we finally reach our destination, not only are we happy but our hearts are light and filled with gratitude and love to share with others. We are better in tune with the infinite.

As I embarked on my journey to manifest my dreams and fully live with purpose, I've been faced with many hardships and barriers along the way. We often think that our dreams are unattainable for this very reason. When we see obstacles in our way, instead of having the courage and faith to strive all the more, we often fall victim to fear and our own self-doubt. Fear is an illusion. The things that we fear most in life only exist within the barriers of our mind. We create these false illusions as restraints because not pursuing our dreams is a lot easier than having faith. To go against what we've been taught and indoctrinated to do is often intimidating. Maybe you've noticed the same to be true with your own personal journey.

As young people of color especially, we are encouraged to pursue our dreams only if they fit within the four corners of the box that society, or our family, has constructed for us. By trying to mold our dreams to fit into this box, we succumb to the fear that limits us and we will never reach absolute happiness.

I've completely done away with fear. "Fear and God cannot occupy the same space," I recently learned from civil rights icon and comedian Dick Gregory. Fear and I cannot even be in the same room; one of us will lose. Recognizing my trials and, at times, seemingly negative experiences as truly a part of the journey has shaped my perspective on life and has positively influenced my relationship with self and with others. My fearlessness has inspired those around me to dwell within the same mindset and to set out on their own journeys to self-fulfillment. It has also caused others to place their own fears, like burdens, upon me. That energy is consuming. Even if it comes from a place of love, fear is toxic.

To let others place their fears upon you gives that person the power to control the direction of your dream. Instead of being in the driver seat of our own car, directing our dreams, by taking on the fear of others, we give them permission to blindly direct and steer our car for us. I never want to be in the passenger seat on the road to realizing my dream. I want to drive. Even if I get tired and have to stop for gas occasionally, allowing someone else's fear to drive me is like giving them permission to crash and totally wreck my dream.

We lose sight of our true selves when we let others take control of our dreams. I've learned that as I pursue my deepest desires, I will be faced with many challenges that will test the faith that I have in myself. It will also make those around me uncomfortable because living in my truth requires everyone who comes in contact with me to question his or her own truths and reality; and adjust. It is easy to become distracted and fearful of change but victory is awarded to the one who perseveres and never loses sight of the end goal. We learn and grow the more we struggle; we win. We lose when we submit our dreams to the fears of those around us.

Be patient with yourself. Practice gratitude. Be thankful for every struggle and every misstep. Every time that I have a setback, instead of complaining, I practice sincere gratitude. I've become truly thankful for the adversity and hardship that I've experienced in my life. Instead of using pain as a crutch to stop me from following my dreams, I turn my poison into medicine. The lessons that I have gained and the knowledge that I have received in the midst of all adversity has made me who I am and has equipped me with knowledge that one can only receive through experience. For that I will always be thankful. Gratitude is what lightens our heavy hearts.

Be in tune with the universe. Meditate. Meditating and chanting has allowed me to find peace of mind. Some of us don't know what we want in life or from our lovers because our mind has not been quiet long enough to tell us. By being in tune with the universe, we uplift ourselves. I can no longer operate on low levels or dwell in dissatisfaction because meditation has allowed me to elevate and understand the oneness of self. Jay Electronica's *"Better In Tune With The Infinite,"* is a song that has helped me on my personal journey. Sometimes the best we can do for ourselves and for those around us is to distance ourselves, whether physically or mentally, so that we may be better in tune with our dreams and with ourselves to manifest infinite possibilities.

Only then can we know peace and love and then, and only then, can we share it with others.

May 27, 2015

With a profound sense of gratitude,
I celebrate my 25th birthday.

I've arrived at a place of peace and love
and appreciation to everyone currently present in my life.
I pray the universe continues to protect me
and guide me in my journey to fulfill my destiny.

My hope for my 25th year is to master self and show love—
to radiate peace.
To let go of all the bad habits
and character traits that has been indoctrinated within me.

Make me whole.
Use me.
This year will be the best yet.

Make me like water.

If I didn't read *The Alchemist* (by Paulo Coelho), if I didn't have maktub tattooed on me, if I didn't practice Buddhism…I may have given up long ago, like most people I presume who live monotonous robotic lives that lack substance, passion, and love. It's been a crazy journey since I arrived in Chicago.

I thought I'd spend my time writing all about my life and how I've evolved in DC and how everything fits together, but I'm still very much living everything that I intended to write. How I expected the story to end, is still being written. Still being lived. I've learned so many lessons in Chicago. The most painful ones. These last 7-8 months have been like Chicago, brutal and cold. And beautiful in ways that I have yet to find the words to articulate.

I've done everything that I set out to do. Melanin Book Club was successful (as successful as it could be, in my opinion), my involvement and knowledge of social justice issues have allowed so much room for growth. I can put love into words and into action. I learned about relationships, friendships and family. They aren't what they seem. I've learned, for a second time, what sisterhood is and what it isn't.

Now I'm at a crossroads between today and tomorrow. The present and the future. I don't know if I'll be in Chicago or back in D.C. All I can do is trust the journey. Trust that it is all written. All the failures and all of the successes are a part of the journey. I can't take anything personally, because it's really not about me. I am just a small part of a big picture.

Something greater.

God.

October 11, 2015

I'm officially back in Washington, D.C.

I am confident that I am where I'm supposed to be. I want to create here and live here. Love here. I can be free. The Million Man March was yesterday. I've never been so charged with building and starting a family.

With the mercury retrograde ending, I think things have returned to the order in which they belong.

As they should be.

It is written.

Love is a choice.

Happiness is a lifestyle.

MEMOIRS OF YBTRENDSETTER
October 31, 2015 | *The Day Before November*

I've been watching the leaves change colors. Green, yellow, some orange then red as they hit the ground, leaving only the brownness of the bare trees. I can't help but think of how miraculous change is and how natural the universe accepts this change. Without struggle. Without complaint. I can almost hear the willows speak. Learn to let the dead things go, and in spring you will blossom all the more beautifully. With each moon comes a new spring. It's the last day of October and it is so beautiful.

I moved back to Washington D.C. after spending eight months in Chicago, I'm back in this familiar place. This space where I learned to be exactly who I am. This place where I learned to love and I learned freedom. This place I question, constantly this place were I seek, and speak, and be. This place where I am. It is not the physical aspect of DC that I crave, and need; it is my own world. A place where I know I have full control and full responsibility for creating. Love and happiness are states of beings, not feelings, they happen by choice not by chance. By chance, we will struggle in sorrow in this world that we live in. But the choice we each have is to love and to be happy.

So often we get side tracked on the road to our dreams by people who fear dreaming. And because we naturally fear dreaming as they do, we become convinced far too easily, and we run. It was a struggle getting back here. It was painful and it was heartbreaking. It was a cold hot summer in Chicago. Filled with grief, with angst, loneliness, and sorrow. But I made it to the other side, closer to my dreams. I set goals and each one of them I accomplished in just eight short months. I met some heroes. I met people who saved my life, a couple times. I died a couple times and resurrected. I created and manifested. I learned true friendship and comradery.

I am grateful. For every moment of pain, and joy. I am finally right where I want to be. Right here, right now. In the present. Not chasing the past or worrying about the future.

I thank whatever gods may be for my unconquerable soul.

November 10, 2015

Everything in my life is new.

My relationship with Jackson; finally being in a loving and supportive relationship for the first time—I want to set intentions for it—but how?

It's simply to love and support and build.
I'm worthy of everything I'm receiving.
I'm worthy of being wealthy.

I want to use my wealth to create and fund all the projects that I have envisioned and sought to manifest.

I want to learn and perfect the cultivation and selling of medicinal marijuana to help fund Black futures. To better my life and those deserving. I have complete faith in myself, my passion and desire, for my own happiness and that of others around me.

I hope to be more patient, more understanding—over standing. Looking with my third eye first. More daring, bold. Unafraid and less timid.

I hope for a family.

Full Moon | January 24, 2016

Just in time for the full moon, my gohonzon is finally up.
My life is slowly returning to the height of spirituality.
Although it has been a journey and will continue to be one.

Today is the first full moon of the new year.
Which is a great day to set goals for the new year.
2016, undoubtedly will be one of abundance.

Thankfully, I've manifested everything that I hoped for.
2016 will require me to be truly convicted in my affirmations
and completely faithful in the Mystic Law.

Allow me to be in tune with the universe.

Fully committed to my peace and happiness,
 first, then that of others.
Allow me to love completely.
Leaving no part of myself in any shadow.
Bring me fully to light.
Illuminate my highest self.
Let no fear or doubt cloud my mind.

Make me like water.
Fluid and transparent.

Like Water
for Chocolate City.

I'm pregnant.

Complete abundance is what I've been pushing toward,
so for this I have complete gratitude.

I am thankful for my womb for restoring me and my foremothers for
making me in their image. I am thankful for Jackson. I've never loved
anyone more. I am completely at peace with him and around him. We
are in tune. We've made one. Although I've been really tired, and nauseous I'm excited. I love Jackson and I can't wait to start a family and to
have a home. I'm faithful. And happy.

I don't know how or when I'll tell people but my pants are too tight and
my "morning" sickness is too much. Food is disgusting and so is sex. I
can't put anything in me without wanting to gag.

My past is finally in the past–it's only right now...
And the future is looking brighter and brighter.

March 13, 2016

I've been pregnant for 69 days now and have probably cried for each of them. But probably more so recently. For some reason I keep seeing my life falling apart right in front of me. I can't remember the last time I was this sad, depressed even, very, very depressed. I can feel it in my whole body. I can barely eat and I don't even want to write. Not even in my journal. My whole life has been this dark tunnel of sadness that I can never seem to escape no matter which direction I go—no matter which route I take. Just as I get back on my feet, I'm constantly knocked back to the ground.

It sucks being Black + woman + 20-something unmarried and pregnant. I literally feel like a piece of shit. I don't think a baby can save me. From me? From what? I wanted to die this week. I sat on the bathroom floor for an hour hoping I'd die—hoping I wouldn't wake up the next morning. I don't know what's killing me slowly.

I don't think Jackson's happy with me. Only happy that I'm keeping his baby. I think he's embarrassed by me, that I'm nothing. That I'm worthless. I have no value and my purpose is fading—my light, dim. I've never been more invisible. I think he's cheating on me. And I'm really fine with it now. I know I can't keep running but it feels like my only option. I'm better off alone.

I know that I manifest everything that I think, that I should be positive. Maybe one day I'll be truly able to master my mind—to be free and happy. Maybe one day. Soon perhaps. Before my own demise.

March 22, 2016

Today was one of those days where I was able to take a step back and really evaluate my current life, my job, and where I see myself in the coming months.

It is springtime.

Winter and its gloom are no more.
Everything is new, fresh, and ready to blossom.

As am I.

Today, I am affirming and stepping into my abundance.
I will be a wealthy, world famous writer and poet.
An amazing mother and woman.

A Queen to Jackson.
I will honor mother Earth and use all that she has supplied to be happy and well.

She will feed me and I will become whole—one with the universe.

Pretty Wings.

I am the master of my fate...*it is written.*

Day 78

March 30, 2016

I know that I've been stagnant lately and this week I've realized how dangerous that is to my happiness. I have to overcome my lack of energy and drive that's taken over because of my pregnancy. I have to continue to set good karma and work fervently toward my goals. I have to be intentional about chanting and intentional about my life with Jackson.

I have been scared to reveal all of myself to him even though this is all I've ever wanted. I'm still scared. I pray that I am able to be caring, supportive, and compassionate with him—to build and grow to produce a rich harvest. I want to love him with all of me without any fear or doubt.

I pray for complete abundance in our finances and in our life. I pray that we are able to start our own cannabis business that focuses on the care of melanated people. I pray that I am able to advance my business of supporting youth and their families. And may we all be happy and well nourished.

I pray that I have complete faith in myself so that I may learn to have faith in other people. May all the hurt and anger from my past never again reveal itself in the present or in the future. May my child know only happiness and true joy. I pray that I have faith in the Mystic Law forever and completely.

Experience in Faith

SGI Buddhist District Discussion Meeting | March 26, 2016

My life has been a continuous journey of both hardships and happiness. I started practicing Nichiren Buddhism with SGI in the summer of 2014, after moving from Chicago, my hometown, to Washington, DC.

Prior to moving to DC, my life had been filled with a lot of despair and unhappiness. My siblings and I were raised in a house where our parents fought all the time. Because of this, we were subjected to and witnessed a lot of abuse–physical, mental, and emotional, from our father. Our parents rarely supported us emotionally because they were dealing with a lot of their own issues. Growing up in Chicago was really hard. We witnessed violence on a very regular basis. Before graduating from high school, my best friend had committed suicide and by the time I had graduated from college in 2013, I had lost more friends than I choose to count to gun violence, police brutality, and gang activity.

In spite of all of this, I graduated from college with honors, was the president of my sorority chapter while on campus, and held many leadership roles. I had become an advocate for social justice, domestic violence, and was politically involved in my community: advocating for low-income youth and their families, hosting voter registration drives, and the list goes on. I realized very early that my purpose was to advocate for people, especially youth, who were just like me but who weren't afforded the opportunity to advocate for themselves.

By all standards, I was successful. I had bypassed all the stereotypes that were associated with young Black women from the south side of Chicago, and unlike many youth from my neighborhood, I had survived. However after graduating from college, I realized that everything around me and everything that I was taught growing up, wasn't as it truly was in the "real world." I was offered a job a couple days after graduating, and I was really happy about that. I was doing everything that was expected of me. I was working for the State of Illinois, assisting low income, first generation students (like myself) apply for college and find money to get to college. It wasn't long before I realized that I wasn't really being an asset to these students, but rather, I was helping the State government get more students to sign up for loans and fall into debt.

We were teaching them that if they got at least a bachelors degree, they would make more money than if they did not go to college. While this may be true for a very select group of people, it was not the reality for the Black and Latino youth that we were working with. And I was proof of this. I had done everything "right" but I was still not earning a living wage, half of my income was being taken from me to pay college debt, and I had to find other jobs just to make ends meet. Ultimately, I ended up moving in my father and his new family and was completely miserable. To be a college graduate and still be extremely poor is a very terrible feeling. Everyone around me was struggling and I felt like there was no way out.

During college, I had the opportunity to travel to Washington DC numerous times to lobby at the capital with my sorority and by junior year, I had decided that I would move to DC after graduation. But after I actually graduated, this seemed like a distant dream. I had no savings and didn't know anything about how to go about relocating to another state. Because of my debt I was unable to apply to graduate school, so essentially I felt really stuck. I couldn't find a better paying job and I had no other option but to live in my dad's basement, working long hours and receiving only enough income to get me to and from work. During this time, I started to write poetry and draw, which was my only outlet at the time. I was even teaching drawing classes to 1st graders. The courage that I received from my art, along with the high school students what I was mentoring, gave me the motivation to pursue my own dream of moving to DC. So I did. After a few months of looking for a job, my sorority sister got me a position at the organization she was working with and a childhood friend allowed me to stay in his apartment while he was away. The job was well-paid and I had full benefits for the first time. When I moved to DC, I started to experience true happiness for the first time in my life.

Everything that I needed and wanted came to me very easily. I had found a cute little apartment after a month of searching, and even though I was all by myself and on a tight budget on the first day that I moved in, I was able to get my whole apartment furnished by a nice couple who helped me move everything in. It all seemed so unreal and I had never experienced such kindness as I did in the first 6 months of being in the District. I loved it here and I immediately felt at home. I was very comfortable. Finally experiencing peace, I was even able to meditate for the first time. One day after spending a couple hours in mediation, I had decided to spend the afternoon at the park reading. On that particular day, I was mediating and asking the universe to guide me in my journey and to reveal my true purpose. As I was walking down the street a homeless woman asked me for a dollar, and thinking I didn't have any cash on me, I told her sorry and continued on my way. Halfway down the block, I had found a dollar in my pocket and quickly turned around to give it to the woman that I had just passed. At that moment, I had ran into Debbie and her friend Akshak, who started conversing with me. We talked about meditation and chanting briefly and exchanged contact information. Needless to say, by the time I had reached the corner to where the woman who had asked me for a dollar was standing, she was no longer there.

Not long after that, I was hanging out with Debbie and she was taking me to YWD meetings and teaching me about the SGI. I started chanting right away and felt a strong connection to the people that I had met going to discussion meetings. It truly felt like home. Chanting Nam-Myho-Renge-Kyo was fulfilling for me and gave me something that other religions had been unable to. It gave me peace and taught me how to be absolutely happy, and I was. I had found out shortly after I started chanting that my cousin-in-law, who lives in Virginia was also a member of SGI. We would chant together, have great conversations, and I even attended some of her district's discussion meetings. I was great being able to chant with family. With the support from and care of everyone around me, I received my gohonzon in December 2014.

While I was absolutely happy, things at my job started to get strange. I noticed that my co-workers and supervisors were being racist toward my sorority sister and me. We were subjected to covert sexually charged comments that would have probably been considered sexual harassment. They treated us poorly and was often passive aggressive and rude toward us. Things got bad after awhile and after my sorority sister was fired unjustly, I decided to resign from my position.

Although I was nervous about being out of a job, I was still chanting and I didn't worry. I was still very happy. At that time, my dad had promised to help my sister and me get an apartment in Chicago. I had been chanting a lot for my sister, who had been going through so much during that time, and felt that if I could be in Chicago, we could both be happy and my dad would be able to restore the damaged relationship that he had with us. Although I was sad about moving back to Chicago, I thought that things would have changed for the better, because I was chanting for my family, hoping to reverse our karma.

The eight months that I spent in Chicago was the worst time of my life. I was once again surrounded by despair and unhappiness.

My dad's promise to help my sister and I get an apartment was immediately broken and the job offer that I had upon moving back fell through. I was once again extremely poor and this time, out of work. I continued to chant and attended discussion meetings not far from my sister's apartment. Although I was poor and struggling to find work, I had everything that I needed and was doing everything that I wanted to do. I started my own business, my book club was prospering, and I was even more involved in social justice issues than ever before. I traveled to an amazing conference, The Movement For Black Lives, with youth organizers that I was working with and I gained lifelong friends. I even took a vacation to LA, where I got to see my mom who had moved to California to take care of my grandfather. Amid all of chaos of Chicago, my unstable living situation, and virtually no income I was somehow still able to find happiness.

Through all of this, my ultimate goal was to return to DC. I learned immediately after moving back to Chicago, that I had sacrificed my own happiness for the happiness of others. Instead of teaching them to be happy on their own, I was only being a crutch. I learned from chanting and from activism, that I had to be at peace with myself before I could help anyone else. 2015 was a test of faith for everything that I had practiced in 2014.

Chanting is like the roar of a lion and as long as I continue to chant I will be able to overcome all obstacles. This time around, when I moved back to DC, I chose to pursue love over money. I am in a happy relationship with Jackson, who I met here in 2014, and we are expecting our first child. I am doing what I love, working in the medical marijuana industry and in training to be a doula. I would not have been able to be where I am today if were not for the many obstacles that I had to overcome and the many lessons that I had to learn. And for that, I am truly thankful for Buddhism for giving me the faith and courage to believe in myself.

April 3, 2016

Hey Mama's Baby,

We've probably known each other for a lot longer, but you've been growing inside of me for around 90 day now. And I still cannot believe it. Unfortunately, words cannot describe the way I feel. But because I love a challenge, I've decided to write to you every day so that maybe one day you will truly know my love for you.

I am happy you chose me. I think I've worked my entire life to deserve you. I'm not worried or too scared these days because you will be in good hands. People are already excited about you; telling me what to do, what to eat, and what not but I know already that my womb is the safest place you will ever be. I'm already slightly protective, not wanting any outside influences to harm you before you even make it here. I'm carrying a Black child inside of me and I realized some time ago that there is no higher honor than that. So thank you for choosing me. For catching me before I fell too hard.

I dedicated my life to you a long time ago. I even attempted to change the world for you. I've been fighting and advocating for you before I even thought of the idea of conceiving you. I didn't know it until this very moment, but everything I've done, everything I've studied, read, and wrote, was for you. You are my world now. My responsibility. My purpose, manifested. I smile at plants blooming and trees budding. I rejoice at the coming of every full moon recognizing that we all derive from the same source. The universe is vast and profound, full of life and love but also of chaos and despair. My purpose is to help navigate you through it, leading you to happiness but not blinding you from all the hurt currently present in the world. It is our ability to withstand adversity that makes us truly human, truly alive. I've dedicated my life to teach you and to love you in ways that no one else ever could.

Simply because I'm mama and you're baby.

April 4, 2016

Hey Mama's Baby,

Let me fill you in on life so far. I'm 25 years old, living with your dad Jackson, whose 27. I was born and raised in Chicago, Illinois by my mom and dad (your grandparents) along with three siblings, Muhammed, Patra, and Malcolm. Long story short, I moved to Washington DC after graduation hoping to leave the past back in Chicago. Strange thing is, the past can sneak up on you no matter how far you leave it behind— and there's no place like home.

I met Jackson in 2014 at the Congressional Black Caucus, we became friends and started dating the following year, seven months later I found out I was pregnant and here we are. Life has truly been a struggle, I really hope you know this—I don't want to paint some magical picture like life is all sunflowers and watermelon. It can be really cold, brutally cold, even in the summertime.

I work at a medical marijuana cultivation center, growing cannabis. Which would have been considered my dream job, had it not been for the slave labor and equally degrading pay. But I love gardening. I love cannabis. Your daddy and I are trying to learn the business to get in the industry, and prosper and win. I love melanated people so I'm doing it for us.

I'm also working on youth and family programs and services for people of color. My main goal is to own a bookstore and cultural center to house my social services, focusing on youth and young adults who often get the short hand of the stick. But the future is brighter because I'm working for you now. I'm in training to be a doula also. The education never stops. I have to constantly progress my knowledge in all areas of education and life. When I first found out I was pregnant, I was reading *Invisible Man* by Ralph Ellison.

Can you hear me when I'm reading to myself? Or should I read out loud? I went to the library today. And just started reading *Sassafrass, Cypress, and Indigo* by Ntozake Shange. My reading list is long and forever expanding, like my library. I hope you'll love it just as much; it's freedom. You'll find the best education outside of the classroom and likely within the corners of your own mind and imagination.

You're growing to the size of a peach this week.
Three months is a milestone, Little One.

Oh, and I'm a writer, a poet,
and social justice activist.

At least I think I am.
Sounds nice, right??

Hey Mama's Baby,

Today was rough for me and I apologize if you felt any of that. I am preparing the best possible experience for your birth and so far it has not been easy. I attended an info presentation for the midwives at the hospital that I've been going to but I was not all that impressed. So I became overwhelmed with thoughts of our birth experience not being all that I envision. The reality is, I'll be comfortable having you in the bathtub and pulling you out myself. I've been crying a lot, do you feel that?

Your dad and I got into an argument after that, with my mood swings and his annoyance of it just made everything so much worse. When we fight I feel even more alone and isolated from everyone and everything that I left behind to love him. He is so difficult, as am I, but he will never admit it. Our communication is lacking—it's scary now that we have you to consider—it's not easy to not talk or just walk away. I love him. Every day I hope you won't be a victim of what we had to go through with our parents as children. Black love is hard and even harder when you've never had any example of a healthy, loving Black relationship. We are growing with each other and sometimes growing is a painful process.

I've been chanting a lot more these days. For all of us. I really want to reverse any bad karma before you inherit such hardship. Although I can't promise you a life without pain, I can promise you beauty, and peace and love. I'm also trying to eat more—you are always hungry. And I'm so picky about food. I just cooked some baked chicken breast, whole grain brown rice, butternut squash, and asparagus. I hope you liked it because after that bath, I am exhausted. I'll kiss daddy for you.

Love.

April 6, 2016

Hey Mama's Baby,

I just got out the bathtub and I'm sitting in the bathroom, with music, a candle lit, in my yellow bath towel typing away on the typewriter your dad got for me. Did you like the tacos from District Taco? I know you've been craving authentic Mexican food. I also got some new pre-natal vitamins for us, which I think will be a lot better for us…vegan, gluten free, multi-mineral, multi-vitamin, sounds fancy right?

Tomorrow I'm going to start looking into other birth centers in DC that will suit us. I think it's important to honor the way in which a Black child enters the universe. I need to be able to light incense, candles, play music, and do everything I can to properly welcome you.

Today I thought about being a midwife. We have lots to journey through, Little One. I have another surprise for you, now. I'm revamping my blog to document our journey. I should be thanking you for inspiring me to write again. I had almost given up hope because of all the gloom and violence looming in the lives of young Black people.

The ancestors gave me you just in time.
They sent Jackson to me just in time, too.
They gave me a family when I desperately needed one, when I needed love. The poems I was writing was probably too sad for them to bare any longer.

I'm happy to be dreaming once again.

I can't wait to hold you for the first time.

April 7, 2016

Hey Mama's Baby,

You are growing so fast…I think I'm starting to show now and apparently you're the size of a peach. You've been pressing on my bladder a lot today, I don't think I've ever peed so much in one day. It's a New Moon so we should set some intentions and get some things done. I'm going to put together an eating schedule so that I make sure that I'm eating enough. I get so moody when I'm hungry and I know Jackson is tired of it.

I don't know why I feel so alone in all of this. My mom doesn't call me as much as I think she should and my dad only criticizes the fact that I'm not married. I have no friends. I left them all to be with Jackson and we can't even go two days without fighting. It's hard not to believe that I may have made a mistake somewhere.

Although you are exactly what I want, I'm scared that I won't have a village for you.

I can hear you saying, "well mom, you have to create one!" and you're right.

Give me courage, Little One.

Please, give me the strength.

Please.

Hey Mama's Baby,

I spoke with your grandma today. She's all the way out in California. Where she should be and where I should probably be, too. She is so excited for you, trust me, she is telling everyone that she is about to be a grandma for the first time. She doesn't know your gender and I don't either but she thinks you're a boy. Jackson's mom is convinced you are a girl. It will be so interesting to see who is right. It's funny that their birthdays are one day apart and Jackson's mom and grandma's first name is my middle name. I miss my mom so much. I think the hardest thing in all of this is being so far away from her when I feel like I need her most. It's really hard. I find myself wanting to cook what she'd cook, or burn the same incense that she would burn, and listening to the music that she loved to listen to. A mother's love is powerful.

Happy New Moon. We have to be clear with the universe about our intentions otherwise, we will welcome chaos and confusion. I want to finish writing my first book by the next new moon. It will bring abundance to both of our lives, and a much needed release. We have a story that needs to be told and old pain that needs to be released. I'm writing this for you so that you will never question any part of my life.

Whether you come to identify as male, or female, you must be in tune with the universe and with your ancestors at all times. Black people have strayed so far from out origins that we've accepted a lot of lies that exist in this society. I will never lie to you. You will come out of my womb full grown. I can only live in this present moment and try my best to plan for the future, but it is already written.

P.S. Your dad thought of the name Jehovah, and something clicked in me.

I love you.

April 9, 2016

Hey Mama's Baby,

First, thank you for giving me the strength to make it through work to-day. On any other occasion, I probably would have quit. My job is not easy but I am thankful for the opportunity to grow myself and this medicine for other people. You help me get through the hardest moments.

I want to tell you how lucky you are to have Jackson as your dad. He probably knows you better than me at this point and he makes sure to ask me if I need anything at least ten times a day. He knows when I'm nauseous that I need to eat or when I'm angry I need to sleep. He is everything at all the right moments and he teaches me everyday how to love.

He has taught me how to dream again and he has such high aspirations for us as a family. He wants to take care of us, because he loves me and you more than anything. We can't be so hard on him—these mood swings are ridiculous and he's usually the victim. Let's play nice. He deserves it and he works really hard to make sure we're happy... so we have to do him just the same.

I'm looking forward to the next couple days and reaching 100 days in this journey.

Tomorrow is Sunday, and I have something special for you.

Goodnight.

April 10, 2016

Hey Mama's Baby,

My surprise for you was supposed to be quiet time for us to spend working on this book I'm writing but instead I spent the day up under your dad, which is what the three of us really needed. I twisted his hair today so that he can start loc'ing his hair like mommy. You'll have locs of your own one day. Black people shouldn't cut their crowns.

I also got us an alkaline water pitcher so that we can have the best drinking water…I'll be drinking like a fish now, I know you'll love that. I'm trying to do better at taking your cues and understanding what you'll need when you need it. I'm doing better, don't you think? I think I did good today at being patient with your dad. He tries the best he can and sometimes falls short, but the fact that he tries speaks volumes. An "A" for effort.

Your granddad will be coming to DC tomorrow, and meeting Jackson for the first time. I really don't know what to expect so I guess I'll tell you more about that tomorrow. I'm really working on not dwelling in the past, especially when it comes to my dad and all the pain he's caused me and the rest of the family. No use in hanging on to old trauma—especially now that I have you.

We are coming up on 14 weeks, and Mondays are usually the hardest so let me get some rest tonight. No waking me up, stay off my bladder a little, okay?

Night, night.

April 11, 2016

Hey Mama's Baby,

I feel so present in this moment. Listening to beautiful music and writing to you. I just finished doing gongyo for the eventing, my daily chanting as part of the practice of Nichiren Buddhism. I think you really seem to enjoy it. I announced your presence a few weeks ago as I was sharing my Experience In Faith at one of our discussion meetings. For the first time that day, I remember, with Jackson next to me and you inside of me I felt complete. Whole. Not as if I was lacking or incomplete, alone, but my whole life had lived up to such a peacefully profound and loving moment. I felt whole with the universe, a oneness.

Your granddad flew all the way out to DC to pressure me about marriage and to give me my mail. And I suppose to see how I was doing, if I was happy or in trouble. I think he expected the later. I'm completely happy, baby. I guess you're the only one who truly knows how much I love Jackson. You chose him before I did, and maybe I chose my dad too. Him and Jackson are out right now, at some cigar bar. Can you imagine? I told him he'd better come home with some vanilla ice cream for us. I was craving the homemade vanilla ice cream my Auntie Dennis used to make.

I have everything I need and I'm evolving more each day and I can't express enough gratitude to the universe and to the ancestors who have guided me. Which ancestor are you?

Welcome to Week 14.

April 12, 2016

Hey Mama's Baby,

Every so often mommy has really hard days. I'm doubtful, tired, and sore. Scared that I'm not eating enough or getting enough rest. Days where I can hardly speak without crying or when I'm barely able to raise my voice above a whisper.

Today was one of those days.

Work is extremely tiring, and I'm barely hanging on.

My back and pelvis is in so much pain it hurts when I stand up and sit down. I just want to lay in the bed and cry.

Mommy needs some rest,
and some TLC from daddy.

Hey Mama's Baby,

Can you believe it's been 100 days? I hope you like it there, inside of me. I'm having a much better day than yesterday mostly because I was celebrating 100 days of having you. Today I made some quinoa with celery and mango, it was delicious. And I'm glad you liked it too.

Today, I planned on recording for the blog, but I was in so much pain. My tailbone aches so bad. I thought that it was from the strain of working in the garden but apparently it's you. Your bones are growing, rubbing against mine...causing me very sharp pain every time I stand, sit, or move without thinking of you.

I can't believe I'm having a baby. The pain, fatigue, and the lack of focus is worth it.

I want to tell the world about you.

By the way, your granddad seems to really like Jackson. I'm not surprised, but surely a little relieved.

Let me get some rest now.

April 14, 2016

Hey Mama's Baby,

I just finished reading *Sassafrass, Cypress, and Indigo* and it has me thinking a lot about you. Wondering if you're going to be a boy or girl. I chose not to find out your gender because I don't want the world to place restrictions and expectations on you because of your sex. And also, mommy didn't want to worry about all the trouble that will come with raising a Black girl or a Black boy.

Raising a Black child now, and before now, has always been a struggle. I already have a lot to worry about without knowing…. I will tell you that whatever you choose to be you will have challenges.

I think a lot about what it means to be Black…

To be continued.

April 15, 2016

Hey Mama's Baby,

I guess I'll be writing you handwritten letters until I can get a new ribbon for my typewriter. Which I guess is nice, that way you'll be able to recognize my handwriting one day, as well as my voice, and spirit. I'm sitting here, listening to my favorite song and record, *In a Sentimental Mood* by John Coltrane and Duke Ellington—the best sounds you'll ever hear. It soothes me and speaks the same language as my heart. Perfect for the moment.

Today I realized that I have exactly everything that I've been praying for—you included. I got a new bike today that I can't wait to take you riding on it this weekend. I've already planned a trip on Sunday for us to go chant at the Buddhist center then go to Eastern Market's flea market. I know you've been craving fresh fruit—I'm tired of all the smoothies too. My bike is a beautiful dark green with a brown leather seat and the same color handle bars. I put a wicker basket in the front and installed a bell on the handle bars for your safety. I'm excited for the weekend. We're going to get lots of vitamin D, exercise and relaxation. We can even go to Malcolm X park for the Drum Circle, if you feel up to it.

I wish I was able to finish my thoughts to you on gender last night but I suppose my ink ran out for a reason and that's a topic we can save for later. As always, I'm trying my best for you. I need to get focused and more determined to finish this doula training. I'm much closer to finishing the updates on my blog, and more inspired than ever to finish Like Water for Chocolate City. I'm trying to love in all the right ways and remember to keep my chakras aligned and my ancestors close. This is all thanks to you

Peace and love are eternal.
Mommy

April 16, 2016

Hey Mama's Baby,

I'm sitting in bed writing to you after completely wearing myself out shopping. My pants no longer fit me and my shirts show too much of my growing stomach. That's all you. We did a lot of walking and got a lot of sun, finally. I'm always wandering out by myself so it's nice having you for company. I really don't want to be alone but somehow I always seem to isolate myself. I was wondering if moving back to DC was a step forward or a step back. I'm still not sure. And whether Jackson and I will be good together, that I'm still not sure of either. I know that with pregnancy comes hormonal mood changes that may make me a little irrational but I wonder. I question, if I'm really happy. What makes me happy? I don't have many, if any, friends out here and no real support system any where. I feel like I'm doing all of this on my own. I don't think Jackson understands or even recognizes this. And the fact that my dad likes him actually makes me nervous.

I'm tired and we're not married, which means I have no security and I can't put all of my eggs in one basket. I have to be self-sufficient, for you and me, especially. We will get there and one day all of these worries and concerns will be memories of the past. I want a home for you to grow up in. For us to love in, create in, grow in. For us to be happy and at peace. This is all that I want. A home to flourish and sustain us. That is something I've never had but always dreamed of. We have to manifest this, by any means.

P. S.
I've been doing a lot better with being mindful of my thinking so that you only hear positive thoughts. Can you tell?

Love,
Mommy

April 17, 2016

Hey Mama's Baby,

I spent all day outside and it was wonderful. For the first time, I felt like I was free, since being back in DC. I rode my bike, got some sun, and saw a beautiful Black family planting flowers in their front yard and I thought of you, of us. I also realized how different me and your dad are.

He'd rather go to a bar or watch sports on a Sunday, and me—Sundays are for praising the Sun and being one with nature. It's scary. I feel like a strange person in a foreign land. It seems like I'm the only person who acknowledges the moon. I have no one to breathe with. I'm alone on a bicycle for two.

We went to Malcolm X park, my spot. They have a beautiful drum circle every Sunday and Jackson couldn't remember the last time he'd sat in a park. How did the universe bring us together? He's experiencing a whole new life with me and I feel like I'm not growing because of it.

I just want to feel home somewhere.

In my 25 years of life, from California to Chicago to DC and everywhere in between that I've lived, I've never been at home. I would argue that it starts in the mind first, so I guess I have some work to do.

-Mommy

April 18, 2016

Hey Mama's Baby,

I think I eat more hot food now that I'm carrying you. You really like spicy things, don't you? Anyway, it's late and your dad is sleeping and I probably should be too. But I spent about a good two hours cleaning this studio apartment that we're in because I couldn't stop sneezing. I like things to be spick and span or I can't think, eat, sleep, or write. So I'm up. I took a bath and now I'm eating—spinach with strawberries and grapes, with chia seeds, broccoli and cauliflower, and I'm trying to decide if I should eat this steak taco from earlier or just call it a night. I hate waking up in the middle of the night hungry. This morning Jackson and I meditated and chanted together. Which is how we should start each day. Every day is a journey.

Congrats on 15 Weeks.

Right now, you're the size of a lemon, or a navel orange. Hair is growing on your head and you may even start to suck on your thumb. I wish Jackson was following your journey as closely as I am. He's excited—but more so about having someone to pay video games with. We had a little debate about it. I'm not against video games, it's just so much to see in the world I'm not sure why anyone would choose to sit in front of a TV glued to some violent game. A senseless waste of time. Learning is so much more fun. I can already tell that our style of parenting is going to be just as different as we are. I just hope I won't be cleaning up after two children instead of one.

I was thinking a lot today of the role of women in the family. We're the keepers of the culture and tradition and I couldn't imagine what life would be like if that weren't so. Jackson had no idea of Black/African culture before he met me, or at least it seems that way. It's women that teach men how to be men. We will see which side you choose. The teacher or the student?

112

April 19, 2016

Hey Mama's Baby,

Today I decided to take a couple days off work to get some rest. I've been straining my back, carrying 5 gallon buckets of water and trying to keep up around the garden. $13 per hour for all that hard labor is hardly worth it. Your dad and I really need to figure out how to grow our own and get moving on starting this cannabis business.

I spent an hour chanting today and it was much needed. There are people that care about our well-being and are chanting for our health and happiness. The three of us will be alright, I promise. I showed your dad some natural birthing videos and he really likes the idea of a water birth. I'm faithful that somehow, some day, everything is going to work out—because we love each other. Daddy just got a new job and is doing well in law school. And soon, hopefully, we'll be moving into a bigger place.

Anyway, I hope you enjoy resting and growing and I promise not to try to do too much. I really wanted to take a few days to get back in the groove of writing and finishing this book—so thanks for giving me a reason and time to do that. I hope, one day, that you'll be proud of me.

One day, I will win awards for my writing and sell millions of books. I will inspire Black people to see beyond their struggle and hope for a better future, better homes.

And we will eat very, very well.

April 19, 2016

I'm 15 weeks pregnant and currently a little nauseous.

I feel so alone in this process although I know I'm not the only young Black mother experiencing these exact same things at this exact same moment.

I have no friends, no sisters, and no support system.
Folks don't even know that I'm pregnant and I wonder if I'm the one that's ashamed and hiding it.

Unwed Black women don't get told congratulations.
We get asked if we're keeping it or not.

I don't think Jackson is ready for any real responsibility.
Am I even ready?

I pray that I am able to manifest energy into telling my story, and documenting every part of this journey for me and for us.

April 20, 2016

Hey Mama's Baby,

I'm doing my best to keep from getting sick. Yesterday I made some tea with my special mix of cayenne, mullein leaf, and lemon to knock some of this out. I want you as well as possible.

Did I tell you how big my stomach is getting? The only pants I fit into comfortably are overalls and leggings. So I will be in dresses mostly for the next couple of months. Enjoy the breathing room—sometimes I have to stop myself from holding in my stomach because I'm so used to it.

Every time I look in the mirror, I realize how fast these days and weeks are passing. Soon it'll be too obvious that I'm carrying life. And I am actually looking forward to it.

The whole world will know about you.

I'm going to give birth to a free baby.

April 21, 2016

Hey Mama's Baby,

I'm lying in the bed—with a headache, my sinuses are all messed up and my body is worn out. Am I doing too much? I swear I'm trying my best to take it easy but even that is too hard to do.

Happy Full Moon.

I want to use this energy to manifest Like Water for Chocolate City.

To manifest a future of financial wealth, prosperity, and complete abundance.

 I align myself fully with the universe to receive all that is written.

A beautiful, healthy baby and family.
A self-sufficient life.
And successful and inspiring writing career.

Asé

Hey Mama's Baby,

It's honestly felt like one continuous day. One long day, with two sunrises and a full moon. I know you've probably felt it. I haven't been feeling good this week and I hope I haven't caused you too much stress.

My granddad died toady. (and Prince died on Thursday)
Everyday just seems more and more foreign when people you admire or love the most are either dead (ancestors) or not yet born (you.)

I wonder what I'm doing here. I was looking up at the full moon, just wishing to be it.

I'm listening to Prince's song *7* and wishing that I had the power to birth you into a world filled with love—not hopeless tragedy, which is what life sometimes consists of. I can't believe my granddad died and I'm all the way in DC. And honestly I have no idea why I'm here.

I wish I was with my mom. I wish to see her and be with her everyday. I feel like a stranger and what's worse is going to be calling her tomorrow and not being able to hug her. I have no idea what I'm doing.

In one month, I will have no insurance and right now I don't have a dime to my name.

Jackson and I are complete opposites and it's really stressful. I don't know how long this will last and I can't help but think of this as some cruel game. Because, what is life?

The odds are against me and I'm trying my best to not give in to depression, but everyday I feel more vulnerable and weak.

April 30, 2016

It's such a strange world, especially when things don't go the way I plan them.

I have no idea what I'm doing here or with this pregnancy.
Things aren't the way I thought they'd be back in October.
Jackson has a new job, so with that and classes and him going out drinking, I've hardly seen him this week. Awkward moments when he tries to crawl his dirty ass in bed at 2am.

I may have made the biggest mistake ever and that sucks.
His mom criticizes my hair and my job and has a tight leash around his neck that he doesn't seem to notice. I pray that I can get out of this situation.

He calls be Q, supposedly for queen, but I think it's because he can't see me for who I am. He doesn't know *me*.

What's worse than being in a relationship with someone who doesn't know you.

Kat,

After giving it some thought, I've decided not to continue at DC Growers. Since I will only be given a floater position and will not be able to finish training on the processing side, there is no benefit in me staying and doing the extra labor while I am pregnant.

Thank you for the opportunity to work with you.

Best,

Melanie

two

On May 10th, I resigned from the position of junior gardener at DC Growers. I started working at DC Growers on December 8, 2015. In this position, I was required to go through a six-month training period where I was supposed to complete daily tasks in the garden and learn different aspects of cultivating medicinal marijuana. On my first day of training, I was given a checklist of things I was supposed to accomplish in the 3-month training on the gardening side of the cultivation center, and after that I would be trained for 3-months on the processing side of the cultivation center. I was never given an official outline of my job description but as it was explained to me, I was to complete the daily checklist and any other assigned tasks.

In the first couple months of working at DCG, I would complete the daily task checklists, which included checking the temperatures of the four grow rooms and three cloners, making sure the reservoirs were filled, balanced, and running properly, checking the sprayers on all grow tables for each individual plant, checking the dehumidifiers, changing the filters, feeding the plants by adding necessary nutrients or water, making sure grow lights were working properly. Along with these tasks, I had to complete the checklist form each day and make sure the end of day procedures were completed. If anything went wrong, I had to help resolve the issue, whether it be with the reservoir, or a pump, etc. I also had to do any other task that was assigned. This would usually mean that I would get off of work later than the scheduled time.

By having to complete the daily checklist and other assigned tasks each day, I was never properly trained on the task outlined on the training checklist. After a few months, there was an infestation of aphids and other bugs throughout the garden, and I was required to clean the reservoirs once a week in addition to completing the daily checklist. Cleaning the reservoirs was a strenuous task, and would often require two people or more to get it finished in the time allotted. The infestation also required the use of pesticides and other chemicals. Not only would the reservoirs, seven in total, have to be cleaned each week, the plants would have to be dunked in the pesticide solution and the grow tables and cloners would have to be cleaned. My responsibilities turned into having to clean the garden and again because of this, I was never properly trained on the tasks outlined on the training checklist.

On March 11th, I was not scheduled to work, but was called in because there was a fire in one of the grow rooms. The fire completely destroyed the downstairs bloom room and caused soot to spread from the vents throughout the entire cultivation center. You could smell the fumes even upon entering and soot was all over the plants in each room. Not knowing how bad the fire was until I got there, I was required to use a face mask to help clean the remains of the fire, complete the daily checklist, spray the soot off of the remaining plants. My asthma was starting to react after a few hours of cleaning, and when I notified Kat, I was asked to go outside to help clean the pipes and the rest of the garden material that was covered in soot from the fire. At the time I did not have an asthma inhaler, because my asthma symptoms were only seasonal (in the fall). On March 12th, I notified Kat that I was pregnant and didn't feel comfortable working with the fumes and soot throughout the cultivation center. It was hard for me to breathe and I would be putting my unborn child in danger. Upon returning to work on 3/14/16, the soot and fumes were still in the air and bleach and other chemicals were being used to clean up after the fire. I continued to work using a face mask to complete the daily checklist and cleaning the reservoirs and cloners. That same day, I spoke with Jon Vincent, the owner of DCG, who said that he would do anything to accommodate me until I was to go on maternity leave and could return after having the baby when I felt ready to.

After that the task around the garden became more difficult and strenuous. My asthma continued to react in the environment and I began to develop a cough from the soot still lingering in the air. The plants had become infested again and we started to use more pesticides. On April 1st, I spoke with my OB at the time about the danger this might cause the baby and he suggested that I reconsider working there because I would be putting the baby at risk largely because of the fire and the pesticides. I decided to work until my six-month training was over, because I would be soon training on the processing side, which was a lot

121

less physical labor. In the weeks to come, a new roof was being added and paint fumes were admitted throughout one of the grow rooms that I had to work in daily. Paint is another risk to women during pregnancy. Soon after, I started to develop severe lower back pain from carrying 5-gallon buckets of water up and down flights of stairs, and constantly bending over to clean the numerous reservoirs, picking up jugs of nutrients and pesticides, and dunking, cleaning, and standing for hours at a time which is not recommended during pregnancy.

In the month of April, I called off several times because of nosebleeds, severe stomach cramping, and mentioned to Kat that I was straining my body too much. I informed her of all of this via text message on multiple occasions. On April 26th, the severity of my back pain worsened to the point where I could not walk, stand, drive or sneeze without being in excruciating pain and was not able to work for two weeks. I emailed my doctor and he suggested I try massages and other techniques, which did not work. I also had to request a prescription for my asthma, which continued to worsen to the point of a mild asthma attack at this time. The symptoms I was facing I thought to be a normal part of pregnancy as a first time mom, however, I later realized were a result of the strenuous hard labor and the hazardous work environment at DC Growers, especially after making my pregnancy known to management. Because it is illegal to fire someone because they are pregnant, I believe that I was forced to work long and hard tasks to drive me to quit.

Not only was the work environment an extreme hazard to my health and that of my unborn child, I was often cursed out by Kat if a task was not done to her liking or if I was unable to complete a task on time. There were multiple instances where hours were cut off of my paychecks. Upon returning to work on May 9th, Kat notified me that I would not be continuing training because I would be going on maternity leave at the end of summer and they would need someone to work the processing side. At that point, she reassigned my duties around the garden to demoted tasks such as helping other employees, washing dishes, and completing some of daily checklist and watering plants.

Due to the fact that I was at DC Growers for over 5 months and was not given the opportunity to complete the 6-month training, the hazardous work environment, and the hard, strenuous labor, and the hours constantly being cut from my paychecks, I decided that it was no longer worth the effort to stay employed at this establishment.

May 12th, 2016

I wonder if the state of my life
is a result of my thinking, past, or inherited karma,
or just lack of effort.

I keep finding myself in situations
where I barely have money to eat,
let alone pay bills.

An endless cycle of depression.
And most of the time I find this world
simply unfit for me to live in,
let alone raise a child.

I'm always hungry with no money and a lot of dreams.
Dreams of being a writer, traveling, helping communities,
raising children and dreams of being free.

But what are dreams? Fantasies?
False realities that will never come true?

I pray for financial security, financial abundance, and financial wealth.

A house, land to grow food and raise children.
To nurture a better society and shape a new world.

May 19th, 2016

"If you change your thinking, you'll change your life."

Today is Malcolm X's birthday
and as I reflect on the life of my ancestor,
I can't help but be thankful.

June 9, 2016

Hey Mama's Baby,

It's been a while since I wrote to you, and with good reason, I promise. The last time I wrote, I started having really bad tailbone pain and
round ligament pain and I was extremely tired. And probably miserable. I started to hate working at that cultivation center and I could tell
it wasn't good for either of us. But thankfully, a lot has changed since
then. I'm not working anymore, I have the occasional back pain but
that's nothing a little rest and a heating pad won't fix. Constipation and
hemorrhoids is a whole other thing though, but no less a part of the process of creating life, which is you. I'm writing you today because I love
you so much. You make me so happy and so hopeful for the future. I
can't wait to hold you. Every time you move around and kick, love just
washes over me. I poke you and you kick back in that same spot which
could only mean that you are just as excited to meet me.

We are halfway through our journey together. Halfway. I pray that I
carry you for a full 42 weeks. I want you to be prime and ready in October because we have a lot to face and learn in this world together and
you must be strong. Yesterday, I had a check up and the midwife took
my weight and measured my stomach. 112lbs and 22in. We are perfect.
You were moving around excitedly and your heartbeat was strong. I am
so proud of the little person you are growing to be.

Walking in to motherhood, for me, has been an interesting journey. But
I am not alone. My cousin, Riah, is 22 weeks, like us and my friend Jada
is 20 weeks. Women are magical beings and I am happy to be experiencing motherhood at the same time they are. I admire them so much.
In the time that I didn't write, a lot has changed. Mother's Day came
and went, as did my 26th birthday in May. Both of those days, my mind
was filled with thoughts of you and my heart was overflowing with gratitude for you turning me into more of a woman, a mother.

I am learning that there is nothing more precious or more powerful than motherhood. I have pictures of both days to show you how you were growing in mommy. You are my sunflower, and I am your Sun. I hope that you will always turn to me and I promise to always radiate the brightest light to guide you, to love you, and to keep you warm.

You are me and I am you.

I've made to grave sacrifice for you, but none compares to the ones that I will make in the future. You are a Black child. Whether male or female, masculine or feminine, your struggle in this world will be no less apparent. But with me you will be more than prepared.

I chant every day for our success and happiness.
For love and health.

With overflowing abundance.

June 13, 2016

I am 23 weeks pregnant.
I am struggling to finish a book I've been working on forever (2 years.)
I can't focus.
I miss my mom, my sistagirl, and my friends.
I'm lonely.
I have heartburn, constipation, hemorrhoids.
I'm probably depressed.
I want a house.
I want to be able to chant, meditate, write and be.
I want to live.
I want to live my dreams.
I want what my ancestors deserve.
I want what my mom never had and what she doesn't know she needs.
I want freedom.
I want to breathe without chem-trails and eat without GMOs, drink without fluoride.
I want solitude and community
I want to be what the universe once was and is dying to return to.
I want to be like water.

2016 Goals:

- House- Home Ownership
- Doula Practice & Family Life Education
- Write Like Water for Chocolate City
- Happy, Healthy Child & Childbirth

I release all disappointment from my mental, spiritual and emotional body because I know that spirit guides me and love lives inside me. -India.Arie

June 13, 2016

Hey Mama's Baby,

Today I woke up and cried for two hours because I miss my mom. I never thought it would be this hard carrying a baby without my mom close to me, to tell me what to do, what to cook, and when to go to sleep (even though I already know.) Still, it sucks. I miss my sistagirl and my homegirls. I've been trying to get out the house more, go on little walks, read out in the courtyard, but for some reason I don't feel safe now that I have you with me. I don't want you breathing unclean air or feeling negative energy. I can control what you are exposed to now, but soon you'll be here and you'll see it and you'll feel it and you'll sense it all. The safest place you'll ever be is inside me, and I'm in no rush (and I hope you aren't either) to bring you earthside. I can wait the whole 42-weeks and be perfectly satisfied.

I'm sitting here watching your dad watch the NBA finals and I hope that you won't like sports. I hope you'll see it as a distraction to what's going on in the world and would rather read a book or write or paint. I wonder what type of person you will be. Who you will look like. How free you will be. I hope that you question everything, and then not be satisfied with the answers that you are given and have the will to seek alternate answers until you find comfort in knowing all view points, all philosophies, all theories.

Tomorrow is the primary election in Washington D.C., and I am going to vote for Bernie Sanders. I wholeheartedly believe that he is the best candidate that this country has for president, and if he doesn't at least win the democratic nomination, our whole world will shift in a negative direction. Hillary Clinton and Donald Trump are both of the same agenda, to keep America, as it is, uneducated and hungry. At least with Sanders, the majority of the country, low-income, young, Black, and Latino people will have a chance at a brighter future. You will. As much as politics shouldn't matter, as free as we all really should be, here in this country it matters deeply and it has mattered for a very long time.

I want peace. And I want happiness for all people.

Everyone around the world is suffering because of this country's indiscretions and political greediness. As human beings, we are all guaranteed the right to the basic necessities; food, shelter, education, health care. And we are all in some way, lacking these in the most desperate ways.

I want what's best for you, always, but I also want what's best for me.

I have dreams that I have to accomplish, that I hope for you to be a part of and hold me accountable for reaching. You are a step in the journey, not the final destination. Together, we will conquer and rule. We will succeed in changing and challenging the world around us.

Thank you for choosing me.

Love,

Mommy.

June 20, 2016

Hey Mama's Baby,

It is the summer solstice and a full moon today, which is extremely rare and extremely special. This past Wednesday, we had a sonogram/ anatomy scan to check that you were healthy. We asked the sonographer to not tell us your gender, because, like I told you, we were waiting for birth to find out. Well, the OB-GYN who filled out the ultrasound results with your weight and everything, checked the box that you are a boy. Completely ignoring our wishes.

I actually wasn't surprised considering how rude and inconsiderate most of the doctors have been throughout my pregnancy thus far. I never knew how disgusting and unprofessional the medical field is, until I got pregnant. They force us into taking tests and try to persuade us to get vaccines, constantly scheduling appointments so that we can keep coming back and they can keep getting money. The whole thing is quite sad. Not only because I've had to go through it, but because many other women have similar, and worse experiences.

Thankfully, you're healthy. That same doctor told us that you were and she also planted a couple seeds of doubt, forcing us to take a blood test to check for genetic abnormalities. I'm confident that you are well. And even more confident that she wanted to not only scare us into seeing her again, but to pay to get labs done.

Fast forward to Sunday, yesterday, was Father's Day and your dad was happy to find out you are a boy. Of course. I'm happy too, but we are happy for different reasons. Men want to have sons. I think some women do too. Girls are seen as inferior and in some parts of the world, are killed for not being a born a boy. I think people will love you more because you are a boy and also hate you because you are a Black boy.

That is the world that you are being born into. Some people will want to see you succeed, and others will make it ten times harder for you to do so.

Luckily for you though, I am your mother.

I enjoy your kicks and punches. They are so cute. You move around so much and it really makes me happy. I've been praying and chanting and hoping to manifest abundance, financial abundance, for our little family. I want a house for you to grow up in, for you to experience the richness of life without having to worry about the color of your skin.

I want to be free, and I want that even more so for you.

This full moon, like the last one, I want financial abundance and wealth. I pray for abundance for you, that you will have everything you will need and more. I want you to have what I didn't. Love and abundance. I hope to finish my book and writings to be able to provide for myself, and you.

I manifest full financial abundance and wealth
for myself and for my baby.

I intend to release all negative and hurtful memories
from my past to have an abundant and healthy future.

I manifest a house for myself and my growing family
so that we may be self-reliant and productive
with what the earth has provided us with.

I pray that I am able to use the energy of the full moon,
the spirit of Nam-Myoho-Renge-Kyo to manifest
my enlightened self and to maximize my highest potential f
or the good of others and myself.

June 24, 2016

Revolutionary Motherhood

- Doula Services
- Birth Education
- Placenta Encapsulation
- Prenatal Yoga
- Homemade Infant Food Recipes
- Nanny/Babysitting
- Woman Empowerment
- Full Moon Manifestations/ Rituals
- Herbs/ Tea
- Cannabis
- Journals/Shirts/Bags
- Literature

I have everything I need to live abundantly.

I am enough

I have everything I need.

Happiness is a choice.

Money does not equal happiness.

I am open to receiving abundance and love.

I am everything I need to share happiness.

I am the Universe.

New Moon | July 4, 2016

What is it that you need to purge in order to make room for the new coming in your life?

So much of my past is constantly reoccurring which shows me more than ever that there are things, memories, and bad experiences that I still need to work to overcome before the baby arrives; most of them have to do with hurt from men and abuse from family.

My intentions for the month are to build stronger relationships with friends and family. To really chant to overcome the karma that we've inherited. I know that I can be distant and difficult but its more import-ant that ever to have strong bonds and roots.

My intentions are to blog about my experience to connect with friends/family who may feel disengaged from me.

My intention for July is to learn gongyo and to share my Buddhist expe-rience with friends and family.

My intention is to focus on kosen rufu and open myself up to abundance and love and care which is what I (and baby) need most.

My intention is to really create a family with Jackson, the family I've always dreamed of having, creating a new future and good causes for better karma.

Happy New Moon.

July 10, 2016

I'm not sure why this baby chose me or what lesson I'm supposed to learn from all of this. I feel sad most of the time and I'm really not sure why. I try to set goals, like my writing, my book club, my blog, but I can't stay focused or encouraged enough to get through it.

I'm constantly wondering what my life would've been like if I had stayed in Chicago.

Did I really chose love? Or did I give up on my dreams?

Jackson tries but I don't think he loves me.
He loves the idea of having children and a family but I don't think he ever imagined he'd be with someone like me. Someone he can't show off; someone who isn't superficial and materialistic. We didn't know each other well enough, now we're in this situation that we can't get out of. He's ashamed of me. He just wanted a baby. And now we're here.

I'm so embarrassed and so, so far from home.

I'm ashamed of me too. I'm disgusted in myself for giving up, for letting go, and it's harder everyday not to let it all go completely.
To die.

July 15, 2016

I suppose now that a part of me is dying and my wishing and thinking of death as something physical, is more of a spiritual dying. Like a new me is being created, along with the baby in my womb. My Self as a creator, as a mother is being developed in my womb. I don't know if Jackson and I will be together long term and maybe we aren't supposed to be.

There is still so much that we don't know and don't understand about each other but all I can hope for is the present. To me, he is the epitome of man. His ego drives him and he is affected by the society he lives in and when things don't fit into society's box, he gets angry and it's usually women (me) that feels his wrath the most. I'm not from here and I'm not happy here and I want so badly to go back to where I became.

I'm not perfect but I strive everyday for perfection; to be as much like The Creator as I am allowed. Perhaps I'm failing and my despair is a reflection of that. I have no wealth and no material possessions of great value. The more knowledge I seek, the less I have. Maybe my karma is too terrible to change to good. I've spent my whole life serving others and have nothing in return. Maybe my smile and my heart aren't worth as much as I thought.

What will I have to teach my son about this cruel, dirty world?
What will I have to show him?
What have I learned to pass down?

Everything I touch crumbles
like dirt between my fingers.

27 weeks/1 Day

1. I'm 27 weeks pregnant
2. Braxton Hicks hurt like hell
3. There's never enough fruit to eat
4. Water isn't supposed to have fluoride
5. I can't chant when I'm depressed
6. I have no friends
7. Suicide is always an option but I lack the courage
8. Men hate feminists and never want a woman who speaks
9. I've been silenced
10. A part of me is dying
11. A part of me is growing
12. I wish I was a bird
13. I hate humidity
14. I should be reading, studying
15. Is love worth it?

Moving Forward | Black Love, Motherhood, & other works of art | July 16, 2016

It has been a while since I last wrote anything on I AM MELANIN, and even longer since I've written anything personal in this space. & for good reason. It's interesting the twists, turns, and the overall journey life brings you on just to get you back on your original path.

I AM MELANIN started off as a blog where I shared my personal experiences as a young Black woman, the things I experienced, and my outlook on the atrocities that were happening in this society and the community and world around me. Soon after, it turned into a place where I offered support, resources, and knowledge to other young Black folks through Melanin Book Club and the array of other services that I wanted to offer to marginalized communities, particularly Chicago, completely taking myself out of the blog all together.

I've learned a lot in the past two years since starting this blog. By choosing to not share much of my life on social media (via I AM MELANIN, Instagram Facebook etc.) I had the space and time to reconnect and refocus. My time of introspection taught me a lot about myself and allowed me to reflect on many aspects of my life and relationships with friends and family. It allowed me to see things from an entirely different and fresh perspective that I admit I was lacking some months ago. I am someone who is always focusing on the bigger picture of society and often have to remind myself of my inner being, where love and peace must derive first in order to radiate outward and have a lasting affect on others.

We have to be really conscious of how much of ourselves we give to other people, whether that be our energy, our time, our body, or material possessions. I devoted a lot of time trying to impact change, to advance a movement, or start one, that focused on helping to resolve issues in our community. I gave up nearly everything that I owned to provide service to others. Which I realized is similar to how I am in personal relationships. I've often found myself in situations where I was always giving time, support, resources to others leaving me completely depleted, defeated, and receiving little in return. It took me a year of struggles and deep reflection (and a lot of people dogging me out) to withdraw from many toxic relationships. The best, and maybe the only way, to remedy issues within the Black community it to start with oneself, your own heart, your own family and friends. As I've been learning more and more recently, there must be a duality and balance in self-care and the care we give to the public.

I spent the majority of my time last summer interacting with and hearing the narratives of young Black people, activists, organizers, students and artists from Chicago and all over the States. It opened my eyes and heart to the overall diversity of Black lives, especially youth, and the deeply rooted individual and communal problems that we as Black people are often shackled by; be it a physical, mental, or emotional bondage, that stops us from living happy, fruitful lives. We end up being on the losing side, constantly in a reactionary mode, and always on the defense. We lose sight of ourselves often forgetting to move forward in our own personal journeys. We remain complacent and silent. Strickened by helplessness, hopelessness, and sometimes despair. I was trying to balance working part-time at a small independent Black school for 2 to 8 year old children on the south side of Chicago, a transitional shelter for teen boys on the north side, building Melanin Book Club in the community and online, organizing, rallying, and community building with various organizations. All of this while trying to build a life and sincere relationships, find stable housing, and have time for myself. That's a lot, even for me, and it takes a lot to truly dedicate oneself wholeheartedly to so many activities, obligations, and expectations without losing sight of something, somewhere.

It didn't take me long to realize my growing need to take a step back to reexamine, refocus, recenter, and restructure the priorities in my life. It is perfectly okay to center yourself in relation to Black Lives Matters. It is okay to focus on the 'right now' instead of what can be accomplished five years from now or some other distant future.

My partner has especially helped me to examine my Self: my biases, my way of thinking and handling racism, prejudice, and sexism and most importantly how these things surface in my own relationships with friends and family. I am still evolving in all of these areas, in all of these ways, and I have learned to adjust my views and beliefs, and overall way of loving and being. I would have never been able to learn all that I have had it not been for having the courage to journey through loving and healthy relationships instead of entertaining toxic ones for comfort and convenience. Perhaps, like I've said and have known for some time, Black love is truly a revolutionary act in itself. Staying alive, staying together, and building a world for our children is what matters most. Living and loving as resistance.

Black lives are intricate. Therefore, we have to be intentional in the way we offer care and healing spaces, the way we educate, and in the way we love. We have to consider every detail, then build and grow from there. Take the time and space to examine the details, the finer, more intimate details that often go overlooked, ignored, or marginalized. I am a better woman because of it, a better partner, and will be a better mother to the life growing in my womb.

This somehow divinely connected and at times bizarre journey through life has brought me to motherhood. When last summer, I confessed that I'd never have children until I was able to change the world around me, until it was safe to rear Black children in communities across the country without them being killed or shackled unjustly. We can't always change the world but we can change our minds. Now when I think of Black Lives Matter, or this movement for Black lives and my place within it, it is not a plea or a reminder to non-melaninated people or to police to cease being racist, to not kill or destroy us—it is a determination, an affirmation, that Black life is prospering in spite of their injustice.

I've always wondered what type of art I would create, what type of businesses I would grow when it was my own children's lives I had to fight to uphold. I've always wondered what type of revolution would brew while I held the life of a Black child in my womb.

It's only a matter of time.

Full Moon | July 20, 2016

140

I don't even know if I should write my doubts and insecurities on paper, if I should keep track of how sad and depressed I've been most days, if I should wonder about why Jackson is always so angry with me-- I don't know if it's even worth it.

All I'm doing is stressing myself out and causing more stress to the baby and at this point--that's my only focus: making sure I'm healthy and happy and the baby is healthy and happy. Anything else is not my concern right now.

I've lived my whole life trying to make other people happy and completely ignoring all of my needs and aspirations. I refuse to keep going down that path.

28 weeks pregnant.

July 20, 2016

Hey Mama's Baby,

I'm so proud of how you've grown and how far we've come together. We are officially in the third trimester, the last three months, the home stretch. I'm becoming more and more excited to meet you, to hold you, and nurture you. I know you're more receptive and your senses are more developed than ever. I've been letting you hear some of your great ancestors and elders speak: Toni Morrison, James Baldwin, Malcolm X, Muammar Gaddafi, and so much more. Can you hear me when I'm thinking? I think you can. I've been reading some Nikki Giovanni and Toni Morrison to you.

You've inspired me to really give the universe everything that I have to offer. And I think you've inspired your dad too. He's following his dream of becoming a pilot. I couldn't be more proud of him. I think he's setting a great example for you, as a Black man, to not fall for the status quo, or do what people say may be best for you. He's following his heart, like you will.

Since it is the last trimester, there are some things that I have to prepare you for and teach you while you are still in my womb. Today is a full moon, and the perfect time to set intentions for the next three months.

I am learning gongyo and chanting everyday.
I am reading *Hey Black Child* to you daily.
I am playing *In A Sentimental Mood* daily.
Positive Affirmations for a positive birth experience, daily. (I hope to bring you in the world peacefully and lovingly!)
Yoga and Meditation: I've been doing yoga daily but I've noticed my need to be in constant mediation is more present than ever.
Manifest a loving village: Reconnect with those that love and support me.

Prepare mentally and emotionally for the change that is coming.
Continue to introduce you to ancestors and elders, educational content,
and nutritious food.

I love you.
I promise to be as calm and positive as I can manifest.
(Although those Braxton Hicks contractions were very painful last week.)

July 22, 2016

Hey Mama's Baby,

200 days. Our last check up on Wednesday went well. You are measuring at 29 weeks, with a heart rate of 142. On Monday we're taking this glucose test to make sure I don't have gestational diabetes. I'm as sick of these tests as you probably are. But I promise, this is the last. And if I can help it, we'll only have one more sonogram. Daddy and I are working on our birth plan at the birth center and we are going to start a parenting group really soon. We're getting ready for you. I'm excited. And scared. Scared that we won't be ready. Scared that the world won't be ready. Maybe I have anxiety at times, and maybe I'm a little crazy. Crazy about what I eat, the water I drink. I try to be positive but it is a crazy world we live in. I promise to protect you and to show you a better life than the one I've known.

No vaccines, cloth diapers, homemade baby food, breastfeeding. It all seems natural to me but for some reason, unnatural in this society. You've changed me. In more ways than one. I've learned what love is through you and your dad. I'm no longer living for myself. I'm living for you. To show you and teach you. And hold you and love you. I can't wait to meet you. To see you. I still can't believe you'll be mine.

It's unreal to think that I could even create and sustain life. Thank you for showing me that. For giving me purpose. I've been struggling to get out of this sad mood, and get out of the house. It was almost 95 degrees today. Maybe it's the lack of sunshine that makes me cry or the hormones that come with pregnancy.

I hope I'm a good mom.

As I'm reflecting on this last trimester of my pregnancy, I'm realizing how far I've come and how much positive energy and abundance I need to manifest in the coming weeks. In 10-12 weeks, baby will be earthside, strong and beautiful, I will be a mother, Jackson a daddy, and we will be in a new apartment--officially starting our family.

Everything that I hoped to manifest last summer has truly come into fruition. I'm living my life the way I've planned to imagine and although everyday is a lesson in itself, I'm truly thankful for every moment, every hardship and every hiccup along the way. Thing aren't perfect, but they are worth it.

This week I will find a Black-owned venue to host our baby shower in September and plan the welcome celebration of love and abundance for out little one.

Jackson will find a good paying job that he will enjoy and that will accommodate his school schedule. My intentions are to set positive intentions for abundance so that all of these things will come into manifestation. May the Gods, the Universe, and the stars align for the three of us.

Happy New Moon.
30 weeks

August 4, 2016

Hey Mama's Baby,

Daddy and I just got back from his family reunion in L.A. where I got to meet so many of his family members and he got the chance to meet my mom and sister, your grandma and auntie. It was a beautiful weekend and I'm happy your dad had the chance to relax a bit. We've been trying to get ready for your arrival and definitely needed to get away from DC for a weekend to help us refocus and recharge.

Last week, I had an appointment with my midwife and she wanted me to take the glucose test to test for gestational diabetes which is common during pregnancy, especially among African American mothers. For the test, they administer a glucose drink and you drink it, wait an hour, and the draw blood to make sure the insulin levels are within normal range. That's great and all and I understand the importance of it but there was no way I was drinking a 10oz bottle of glucose, and who knows what else they put in it. So instead they gave me the alternative of drinking 8oz of Welch's 100% Grape Juice and 1/2 a banana which equaled the same 50g of sugar as the glucose drink.

I'm telling you this because I want you to know how important it is to research what goes inside of your body, your temple. Not all doctors are here to protect your health and well-being, and as a Black person many doctors will do what they've been taught and that is geared toward white men. So proceed with caution and knowledge. The lab attendants definitely tried to insist I drink it, almost forcing me to, but I held my ground for you.

We come from the earth (and one day we will return to it) and there is never a reason to substitute natural for artificial. In other words, holistic health is better than pharmaceutical. I can't wait to teach you these things. I'm teaching your daddy this too and he's grown so much since.

With the passing of the New Moon, I've set positive intentions for your health and well-being. I'm setting great causes so that daddy will find a good job and we'll move into a new home before you arrive.

I am welcoming all forms of abundance for the baby shower to celebrate your life next month. We are at 30 weeks now. 7 months! Can you believe it?

You've done such a good job and I am so proud of how you've grown. My mom said that the best women have boys first, and although I hate gender norms and whatnot, my mom,
your grandma, is always right.

Love you most,
Mommy

August 11, 2016

Hey Mama's Baby,

I'm getting more excited for you with every letter I write, and when I'm not writing I'm thinking about all the things I want to say to you. I'll start from last week. On Sunday, I spoke at the World Peace Gongyo meeting about the importance of sharing Buddhism with others, especially through friendship, and forging true and genuine friendship. There is no reason why anyone shouldn't know that I am Buddhist and practicing Buddhism. I want to be sure to include you in everything I'm doing now because you have been a major cause for growth for me in the last seven months. I have to show you my gratitude for allowing me to go through this rite of passage. I spoke to a room full of people; over one hundred, and many of them were very impressed with my public speaking and the speech itself. I've very glad you were on your best behavior and I felt well enough to get through it. I wasn't even nervous. I was excited to finally be able to get involved with SGI. I have to teach you all about it, but I'm sure you already know the language of the universe.

On Monday, mommy started a new job working with women and their babies. And once you arrive I will be able to bring you to work! It is such a dream job right now and I'm so lucky you helped me get the job. The fact that I was pregnant was a huge plus. They've been helping me already with healthcare and education. You will have a village to grow and thrive in. I've been chanting so fervently for this and I wasn't even thinking of it coming in the form of a job.

Daddy was just offered a job today, working at a casino doing surveillance. I think we've both been making great causes. Jackson has been so receptive and encouraging of my chanting and Buddhist practice. I'm making him plan your baby shower, although I'm micromanaging. We are celebrating at a game room/bar.

In the midst of receiving all of these benefits, my old roommate passed away from stomach cancer. It was incredibly tragic for me because we were good friends throughout college and she was always around to support everything I did. We lost touch shortly after college, I moved to DC, and we hadn't spoken nearly enough. This is the second close friend I've lost and regretted not speaking to consistently.

This whole situation has been an eye-opening lesson, in the importance of checking in on people, family and friends. I think that in time I will work more diligently to stay connected, to build more solid relationships and a stronger community.

I'm chanting for your health, and daddy and I are still battling over your name. I think I won in that it will start with an *M*.

Love,
Mommy.

August 15, 2016

I've always imagined my life just as it is and it is so beautiful to realize. Although many things are still being manifested. I am thankful for everything that is. I am working now with an amazing organization that offers maternity support services to Black women and children (for us, by us) and it is the most beautiful thing to be a part of.

I chanted wholeheartedly for a village for my little one and I found it. I interviewed and was hired on the spot. The universe truly does conspire. We may have even decided on a name and finally sent out baby shower invitations. Everything is falling into place as it should and I will continue to chant, meditate, and affirm everything that's to come.

Tori sent you a private note:

Why would I come to a baby shower for a baby that my "friend" has never even told me she was pregnant with? This is my first time being formally told Melanie is having a baby. It doesn't make sense to invite someone to your baby shower if you have never personally shared with them the news that you were pregnant in the first place. I expect more from a "friend" who I helped welcome to DC in 2014. Who I helped become the successor of the position I was promoted from at the Research Institute; I literally coached her through the interview and they solely hired her based on my own merit at that time. I let her stay at my house, helped her with food, and put her onto my weed man. She also quit the job two weeks after I was fired from the job and then moved back to Chicago in January 2015 without saying a word to me. Nothing at all and I had just saw her...I had to find out from one of our other line sisters that she moved back to Chicago. Last fall I wasn't even fully aware she moved back to DC after the Million Man March until I was told from someone else and we eventually connected again. Overall, I have been a friend to Melanie and always tried to look out for her, but she has not done the same for me. We have not spoken since February and if she wanted me to know she was pregnant she could've called me. Sorry, but no gift from me...

Hey Tori,

You don't have to come to the baby shower at all, in fact, it was Jackson who suggested we invite you. You were, however, the first person that I told that I was pregnant back in January when we met up for drinks and dinner and you were far from supportive. If you look back through our text messages, I was constantly inviting you to hang out with Jackson and I, and you always declined or never got back to me. Then you contacted me to be used as a reference for your job interviews, and I did so twice. I asked you to do a reference for my Teach for America application and you never even completed it. At that point I figured that you were not interested in continuing our friendship so I stopped making attempts to hang out with you, and since you made no attempts either that solidified it for me.

I guess you don't recall how they treated us at the Research Institute, and you in particular. Yes, you helped me get the job, but I resigned after they treated us so poorly, fired you unjustly, and then offered me your position. If I was a bad friend, I would have taken the position and would not have had to move back to Chicago. I expressed my gratitude to you for getting me the position and helping me get adjusted in DC when I first moved here, however, I think you saying I stayed at your house and you helped me get food is a bit of a reach and you know it.

Every decision that I made to move back to Chicago or DC was a very personal one, and I did speak with you about them each time. It was you who suggested that I consider moving back to DC last summer. I didn't tell anyone that I was moving back out here for a few weeks because I wasn't sure if I would be staying, and when I was sure, you were of the first to know. It is so appalling that you would say that I never had your back when that couldn't be further from the truth. I've supported you in so many ways throughout these years and I do apologize if you've failed to realize that. I am not holding on to any negative energy, because it's bad for the baby, and I refuse to live in the past. As always, I wish nothing but the best for you and will continue to pray for your happiness.

Peace,
Melanie

Melanie,

I honestly don't recall you telling me you were pregnant at all. I just remember you telling me that you both were going to look for a two bedroom apartment. Perhaps, you thought you told me then. My first time hearing of it was when our line sister told me this past May. I did not do your Teach for America letter of recommendation because I was contacted by one of the jobs I applied for and they informed me that they heard back from all of my references except you. I then realized how I had helped you get a job and did your Peace Corps letter of recommendation back in June 2015, but you couldn't do a phone recommendation for me. If you did do the phone recommendations, you never contacted me to let me know that you completed them and what job called you. When I did your Peace Corps letter of recommendation, I know I followed-up and let you know it was completed. That is why I stopped contacting you and why I feel the way I feel towards you. It has been a build up since the Research Institute...

You staying at my house and helping you get food is not an over-statement because I did help you the first few weeks you arrive to DC and you know it. How unappreciative and ungrateful you are to downplay it. I would even hook you up with free drinks and wings sometimes when I would bartend. I would also pay for an Uber to your house and you wouldn't even offer to split or put on. Yes, we would smoke at your house, but often times Raymond would come pick me up and blow with us without you having to match. Also, every time we would hang out with Raymond you never had to put up money for food or drinks. He would take care of all three of us, opposed to the one time I hung out with you and Jackson I paid for my own drinks. I don't expect him to pay for me at all, but the difference is my man would even look out for you because you were my friend. So let's not talk about looking after someone, because I can't recall you ever providing me with a place to stay for a week or two. Can't recall you ever buying me food to eat, helping me get a job so I can relocate and have money in my pocket, or pay for me an Uber home.

As far as being treated badly while at work, I don't recall any of the mistreatment occurring before you arrived. Before you arrived I was doing well as an employee, I had stellar performance, great work rapport with everyone in the office, and was promoted with a $10,000 raise. Thank you for teaching me the lesson to never help a friend get a job where you work because it can change the entire dynamics at work. You were constantly late every single day at work (yes I was late too, but you were late so much Lita would come by my desk and ask me was everything okay with you...why because I vouched for you) and you would openly read pro-Black books in their face. Of course they started treating us badly because they probably assumed we didn't like white people. You directly exhibited this behavior and because I vouched for you and helped bring you on-board I was viewed in the same light. I will honestly admit the conversations we had about pro-Blackness and such at the time impacted my work performance and motivation. That's my fault for following your influence, but it will never happen again.

When you left DC last February I was not informed. I remember when I came home late Feb 2015 to check on my mom and I asked you why did you leave so quickly and I didn't even know you were back in Chicago for good. I asked you what did you do with your furniture and everything because I had no idea. After my mom's funeral, I did mention that maybe you should move back because of the things you were sharing with me about your living situation at that time. Plus, when I got back to DC, Raymond and I were driving past Bus Boys and Poets in Brookland one day and it was really busy. I thought maybe Mel shouldn't had left but I never heard a word about you moving back for real until you were already here. So no, you have not communicated with me throughout each time you've left or moved back to DC.

Nonetheless, I wish you the best as well. I also apologize that you don't realize HOW much of a friend I have actually been to you. It's very hurtful to hear you speak to me as if you are the one who should have a chip on their shoulder, when in reality you have not done as much for me as I have done for you. You know what you've done for me does not compare. Anyone I explain these circumstances to gets it...

With pride and respect,
Tori

I'm sorry if you feel that my presence at work caused you to lose your job. When I was late, which was not everyday and not as often as you, I would inform Lita and if she did have a problem she would have talked to me about it, but she never did because it was often the redline train that had delays and that was out of my control and she knew that. Lita and Erika would inquire about you with me all the time, as I told you back then. If my work ethic was ever in question, I would not have been offered your job after they fired you.

For you to blame me for your lack of performance and motivation is childish. I could not care less about what anyone, especially non-Black people, assume from the pride that I have in my culture and I would never try to hide it to benefit them or their companies. I never read at my desk, nor did I ever say or act like I hated white people. I'm sorry if you think I didn't complete your phone references, I definitely did. It sucks that instead of checking with me, you assumed I would do that to you. Anyway, I apologize for the miscommunication. I did tell you, before anyone, that Jackson and I were talking about marriage and starting a family, and you completely dismissed it. But I knew that you were going through a lot and did not hold it against you.

For anyone to keep a list of all the favors they think they've done me, is not a friend or sister to begin with. I also apologize if you feel unappreciated, but that has nothing to do with me. I've expressed my gratitude to you (and Raymond) many of times, but if you think I owe you information about my whereabouts when you clearly have ill wishes towards me is truly asinine. I've been nothing but sisterly to you when very few people wanted to be, because of instances like this.
Please forget that I ever attempted to reconnect with you.

All the best,

Melanie

Aug 15, 2016, 2:58 PM

I didn't blame you I just said that I let your actions influence me at the time. That's not blame, I'm stating what I realize I did wrong. Which isn't childish at all. You're response lets me know that you ultimately don't care about how much I've been in your corner. I mentioned those things to make a point because you can't even send me a list of the things you've actually done for me. If you could, I'm sure you would've replied stating such things instead of expressing how "unsisterly" I am. If I am "unsisterly", I can say the same about you.

Yes, you've told me that you appreciate the things I've done for you, but have you shown it? You as a woman of Delta, my own line sister, know first hand that ACTIONS SPEAK LOUDER THAN WORDS. Your actions have not shown me that you don't appreciate the things I've done as a friend. You really don't have a rebuttal otherwise you would tell me in what ways you've been there for me outside of emotional support from time to time.

It's very unfortunate to have to sever our friendship in this way. I wish no ill-will towards you and many blessings for your unborn child and family. I just hope as you mature you understand how to treat those who have lent a helping hand to you, instead of taking their help as a grain of salt and moving on with your life. Please hold yourself accountable for your part in damaging our friendship and sisterhood.

With Pride and Respect,
Tori

I hold myself completely accountable for my part in ending our friendship/sisterhood, as I said, I am not interested in being friends with anyone who makes a list of things they think they've done as favors to me.

It is obvious that our expectation/definition of friendship is completely different. I value emotional support in any friendship, more than anything else, and in turn have always given that to you, which is what true friendship is to me.

I'm sorry if you feel differently and/or can't see my perspective. I will never be able to send you a list of things I've done for you because that is not something that I was aware I was supposed to be tracking.

Actions do speak louder than words, and my actions have always proven true. I'm always moving upward and onward and will always appreciate your help in my transition to DC.

All the best to you as well.

Well clearly your perception of friendship is to use a person until you don't fuck with them anymore.

Your actions have only shown me that you use people for what they can do for you and you can't even offer the same...

It's cool though...moving on.

With Pride and Respect,
Tori

August 21, 2016

Today has been one that I just don't understand. In fact, these last two weeks have been hard for me to grasp. Jackson and I are in a love/hate relationship that is starting to feel more and more unhealthy. Sometimes I feel like he truly loves and adores me, and other times, especially in front of his family, its like he doesn't know me or want to be bothered by my presence. It's scary to think that I'm having a child by someone who can love me then hate me so easily. I decided to stop having sex with him because I don't feel like we connect on a spiritual level and I refuse to give my body to him--until he is spiritually in tune with me and the universe. He is always angry and I really don't get it. Maybe today was the day where his anger finally got the best of him. He'd been scream-ing and cursing at me all day, grabbed my gohonzon and attempted to damage it. When I went to grab it, he pushed me so hard that I fell on the floor-- on my side. I couldn't believe it and still can't.

I've never been so disrespected in my life. Not only did he try to harm me spiritually, he put both me and the baby in danger physically. These last couple days have been filled with stress and I've been trying to be strong and calm for the baby.

Jasmine, my old roommate and friend, passed away on the 8th and on the 18th was Kristina's birthday and on top of everything, I ended my friendship with Tori. Maybe all of this, of course is happening now for a reason-- karma? Did I somehow deserve this? Maybe that isn't even a question, I do deserve it. I'm such a terrible friend. Everyone that gets close to me ends up hating me for one reason or another. Whatever the reason, whatever the lesson, I just pray that my baby isn't hurt and all of this stress doesn't cause me to have preterm labor. I packed all my clothes and I'm not sure if I will move out yet but I know I'll feel like an idiot if I stay and Jackson gets more aggressive, hurtful, and disrespect-ful.

Tomorrow I will start chanting again because there is no way that I will allow this to break me.

230 Days pregnant; 32 Weeks, 8 Months

Hey Mama's Baby,

I've been meaning to write to you for a couple days now but I think I've been stressing myself out. The mind is truly a powerful thing. It can encage you if you use it incorrectly. Daddy just signed the lease on our new apartment yesterday, and we are moving just outside of DC to Greenbelt, Maryland. It was very hard for me trying to decide on a place to live because I not only have to consider my comfort, but yours as well. But we finally agreed on a place and got the keys the same day. Now begins the process of packing and moving.

Daddy and I were both a little apprehensive about the new apartment. The outside doesn't look all that great. And I was honestly a little scared. It took a long bath for me to realize how we are truly living in abundance and it's the inside that matters most. We can complain, or we can make the best of it and be continuously grateful. So I've decided to be grateful. I am so proud of the man that you'll call daddy. He is working so hard to provide a life for us and he doesn't complain for a second. He loves you more than he loves himself.

Anyway, your baby shower is in 10 days. Can you believe it? I can't. I'm sad that a lot of my friends, family, and sorority sisters won't be in attendance but your dad has a great support system and we will be surrounded by love. This is another one of those things that have tried to stress me out but I'm choosing to be grateful.

This is a new journey for us, all of us. I'm nervous, as any new mother would be but I'm confident, with your daddy, that everything will work out for the best. We've decided on a name for you as well. You kick every time I call out to you. How sweet can you be?

My little prince charming, I cannot wait to meet you. I'm so proud of your growth and I hope you continue to grow strong and healthy. If you do decide to come early, don't. I'm about to start nesting soon.

Love,
Mama

Hey Mama's Baby,

I love you. I just want you to know that.

I can't stop thinking about you and imagining holding you, kissing you, and loving you for the first time and for the rest of my life. I'm a lot more sleepy these days, and quiet.

I know it's time to start nesting and this New Moon (and Mercury Retrograde) has made it much more obvious that we are getting ready for a new phase in our lives.

Daddy is ready to start nesting too. He worked so hard to find a great apartment for us and is at the dealership trying to get a new car for us.

I'm so proud of him and proud of you.

Love,
Mommy.

Full Moon | September 16, 2016

It seems like so much time has passed since I wrote last—so much has changed. Jackson and I just got an apartment in Greenbelt and I can honestly say that I am happy to be out of DC and putting all those memories behind me. This is a new chapter in my life and I want to and intend to embrace it with complete light and positivity. Jackson and I are growing together and I think that is the scariest part of the whole journey—the fact that we are still "getting to know" each other and still growing everyday.

It's been a long eight months and I know that it will be even more difficult when the baby arrives. Nonetheless, I am very thankful for the love that we do share. We still have to learn how to respect each other fully and a lot has to happen before we can even think of taking our relationship to the next level.

Right now anyway, I am focused on making sure I have a peaceful birth experience. I will have the birth that I've dreamed about, and our baby will be happy and healthy.

Messiah Maxwell
36 Weeks, 256 Days
8 Months

September 16, 2016

Hey Mama's Baby,

So much has changed in the last two weeks. Today is a full moon and not only am I nesting and preparing your nursery (yes, nursery) but I am also still working at Mamatoto Village until the 30th of September and taking a hypnobirthing class. We also have a new Jeep, which will be perfect for you and the ride is much smoother than daddy's two-door sports car. I know you're getting ready in your own way and reminding me to slow down, eat more, and drink more water.

We were able to view the birthing center where I will be birthing you and now I know that time is nearing. I'm even more excited about meeting you. Did I tell you about your baby shower? It was last Sunday and so many of our friends and family came out to welcome you.

We also got a lot of gifts, and even more gifts are coming in the mail everyday. We will have a peaceful and beautiful birthing time and I am excited to finally be able to hold you.

Tomorrow we are going to a formal dinner, President Obama will be speaking and I am excited to bring you along for the journey.

Everyday I am reminded to remain calm and positive about birth, without letting anyone's terrible birth story sit in my subconscious.

My body is meant to carry you full term and birth you quickly with little discomfort.

-Mama

September 19th

I am ready and prepared
for my beautiful and peaceful birthing

I see myself birthing beautifully,
calmly, and with confidence.

I feel confident about my body's ability to give birth.

Peace.

I look forward to giving birth
with happiness and excitement.

September 19, 2016

Hey Mama's Baby,

I'm sitting here listening to the rainfall, the rain water hitting the trees, the ground, and the windows. Sound is the most relaxing and comforting thing about nature. I thought this would be the perfect time to write to you. Right now, you are as close to nature and the earth as you will ever be. I hope that you embrace this time in my womb and find peace there. I hope that when you are ready to come earthside you do so with peace and beauty. I wish for your journey to be soft and gentle. Loving.

I can't wait to see you. Each day feels better than the next, knowing that I am one day closer to loving you even more. I will be able to love you with all of me. My fullest devotion and attention.

I named you Messiah. Messiah because not only do you have much to live up to, but you are already an anointed one. There have been many great before you, and you are responsible for the greatness of those who will come after you. So, I am already proud. I adore you already. I sing my praises to the future of our race.

Malcolm
Mandela
Marcus
Martin
Muammar
Messiah.

Love,
Mama

8 Months Pregnant

September 25, 2016

Hey Mama's Baby,

I'm hoping that you get all the rest and nourishment you need for now and I promise you can come out in a couple weeks. The full moon is October 16, just to let you now, that would be a great day for birthing.

As for right now, I'm taking a hypnobirthing class to prepare for the big day, I'll be washing your clothes, blankets and towels tonight, and packing our birthing bags. Tomorrow will be dedicated to cleaning. I'm trying my best to get your dad to clean and unpack his things but he is stubborn and is used to being spoiled so of course he hasn't done it yet. Nonetheless, everyone is excited to meet you and some even think you'll be coming earlier than I expect. You should know that mommy does not like surprises, so if you do decided to come, please let me know.

There is a lot going on in this outside world. The police are unjustly killing Black folks left and right, the statistic is every 28 hours actually. Protests and riots are erupting in various parts of the country. The country is also in the midst of a "very important election" that can and most likely will have a huge impact on our future. Democrat Hillary Clinton vs. Republican Donald Trump. Both candidates couldn't care less about the lives of Black people in America. That we know for sure through the actions of Hillary Clinton and the words of Donald Trump.

Many Black elders are trying to urge us to vote for Hillary Clinton, because she is both a Clinton and a woman but have completely ignored her past actions regarding mass incarceration of our people and that she is also, most importantly for me, responsible for the killings of great world leaders such as Muammar al-Gaddafi, who you learned about a few months ago. For me, I am not choosing the lesser of two evils.

I thought about sitting out of this process and not voting at all, but you have to understand that Black people and women have struggled and fought for the right to vote here in America. To have a fair and equal chance to choose the candidate to represent us, our families, and better our lives. So I may just vote on that principle, maybe, for the libertarian candidate. Or I may just pencil your name in. Because I believe more in you than in anyone else in the world.

Last night I had you listen to some slave narratives. Just so that you'll know the history of where we started in out in this country. Most of our history is lost, and stolen, and given back to us in pieces, lies, and half truths. But mommy is a truth teller and seeker. There is so much that you will have to learn from me that is not currently taught in schools and is hidden in books.

Are you the one?
Are you the one?

Love,
Mama

Week 37 - Day 265

October 12, 2016

Today is Messiah's due date.

I gave birth to Messiah on October 2nd around 1:08am. At home. On the couch. Well, it was more like Messiah gave birth to me. He practically delivered himself.

I am currently healing and experiencing life as a new mother. Having to care for a small human life is a bit of a challenge and probably the greatest responsibility I will ever have.

I am grateful for the wonderful and safe birth experience and I pray the universe allows me to share with other women how lovely giving birth is when we are able to own our experience and not let professionals make decisions for us.

These past ten days have been a journey. Each day presents a new lesson. I gave birth to a beautiful healthy 6lb, 7.5 oz baby boy.

He is brand new. Safe and protected.

October 12, 2016

Hey Mama's Baby,

Today is officially your due date. But you blessed us with your presence 10 days ago, October 2nd around 1:08 am. My beautiful surprise. I love you so much. We've been on a journey for these last ten days, getting to know each other, bonding, and growing together. I am so happy that you are healthy and beautiful. You came into this world peacefully. My peace baby. You have my whole heart and each time I look in your eyes I fall deeper in love. Every time I feed you from my breast, I fall deeper in love.

I birthed you in our new apartment, your new home. Just me and daddy. I think you were ready to hang out with us, and just like that you came. I wasn't in labor for more than an hour. I pushed three times and you came. It was a rainy day, I spent the entire day in your room organizing your things and meditating on my journey thus far. Daddy had a test for the FBI and was gone all morning. We were enjoying the sound of the raindrops. And when daddy came home, we had a long hug and he made lunch. We took a long nap, watched Luke Cage on Netflix . I made brownies and daddy went to get dinner from Chipotle.

We spent two days in the hospital after your birth.

It seemed like the longest two days ever. I was on alert making sure doctors and nursing didn't inject any vaccine into you or do anything to harm you. I hate hospitals. There's no place for Black people in a white hospital. We were are Holy Cross hospital in Silver Spring, with the crucifixion of jesus hanging in our room. What an awkward place for you to spend your first few days. But I think being in that small room, you and I both very vulnerable, bonding with daddy, I believe it made us stronger. A family was born in that room, 4226.

I birthed you and you birthed our family. I am forever grateful.

October 14, 2016

I can't believe I caught my own baby. 12 days postpartum and I'm still in shock. I had no idea how much my life was truly going to change the moment I pushed Messiah out into the world.

He is lying on my lap at this very moment, because if I put him down too soon, he'll yell and want to use my breast to pacify. We spend all day together. He sleeps on my chest or in my arms every night because I guess his co-sleeper isn't close enough. We smell like each other. Most mornings I can't tell if its his dirty diaper or my pad that needs changing.

I wonder what it's like for Jackson to see us everyday. Now I see how easy it is to lose sight of a spouse or lover once a baby is brought into the picture. I hope he loves me through this. Through my "ugly" phase–although motherhood is beautiful, I sure feel ugly. With my stitches and hemorrhoids and postpartum bleeding–it's all a bit much.

Nonetheless, I know that I need to maximize this time. I'll never have these days back and I want to make sure that I record every moment through text.

It's not solely Jackson's responsibility to make sure Messiah and I live well. There is so much that I need to make manifest. And I will.

Full and complete financial and economic abundance.

Love.

10 Days Postpartum

Hey Mama's Baby,

Today you are three weeks and two days old.

At birth, you weighed 6lbs, 5 oz, then you dropped to 5lbs, 15 oz two days after that. I was so worried about you, making sure we were nursing properly.

It's so much moms worry about with newborns that I didn't think to preoccupy my mind with before now.

23 Days Postpartum

October 30, 2016

This month Jackson and I had a baby and are celebrating our one year anniversary. And what a year it's been.

My journey into motherhood has truly been just that. I can't believe today, Messiah is 4 weeks old—just a couple days shy of one month. I'm in awe everyday of this little soul, who chose me to be his mom. I'm not perfect and since becoming a mom—I have no longer the urge to try to be. I can only do my best and be my best.

This month I've learned the importance of caring for myself, my health and well-being comes first. Even before Messiah; so that I am better able to care for him and respond to his needs.

I pray that Jackson, Messiah, and I continue to grow as a family and that we have complete faith in the Mystic Law.

I pray for our health, security, and safety.

Love.

November 2, 2016

Messiah is one month old and I am just thankful for his life.

He is such a wonderful child and I am thankful that he chose me and Jackson to be his parents. Everyday has been a lesson and a milestone. I've honestly felt like I've been in another world.

I love Jackson so much more than I realized and everyday with him is special. Each month will be a new gift and another opportunity to express sincere gratitude.

November 9, 2016

Every day, for more than a year, I've been praying for abundance.

Today I light this candle and do the same. I've received so many gifts, abundance. I pray that I remain in tune with the universe, under guidance from the ancestors so that I may continue to be open to receiving abundance: Everything that Messiah deserves.

I'm sitting here, nursing Messiah, thinking of how I'm responsible for him, his knowledge and awareness. Another generation of us. American Blacks. Black American. African American. Black American Native. What a gift and an honor...

Gratitude.

November 10, 2016

I pray that I am a great mom.
I pray that I am the best mother that I could possibly be.
I pray that Messiah grows into a child of good character; a child of the universe.
I pray that he may be the anointed one.
I pray that he may be a teacher and a student.
I pray for his good health.
I pray that we grow together as a family with love surrounding us, like a bubble.

I pray for my own health and safety; and for Jackson.
I pray that he be genuinely happy.
I pray that whatever career he chooses, may it fulfill him completely.
I pray that he continues to love me fully, with his complete mind, body, and soul. I hope that our relationship will grow into one of loyalty, honesty, and sincere friendship.

I pray that our love will last forever and always.

I pray that I may be able to walk boldly, strongly, and confidently into my purpose. I pray that I attract only light and positive energy. I pray that love may be felt through my energy and through my words.

I pray that my words will move millions of people. I pray that I will be able to write truth and healing words for every soul that may need it.

I pray for complete abundance. May my words and thoughts bring wealth and prosperity. Money and respect.

I pray that I stand firmly with my back straight and my head high. I pray that I am my best person at all times. Always, living and being without ego.

I pray for peace.

Full Moon | November 14, 2016

Today I realized that I'm not the same person I was nine months ago.
I am a mother. I am a new woman.

Everything about me is new; is different.

I pray I use this Full Moon, Super Moon to realign and renew myself.

I pray that my chakras are balanced.
I pray that Messiah's chakras are balanced.

As I continue on the road to learning this new Self, I pray it be gentle
and kind. I'm coming to understand life, love, and family on another
level and I just pray that the universe takes it easy on me.

I pray for abundance and success. I pray that I am able to manifest everything that I have written in this book and those before.

I Am Melanin.

As I am starting to regain my sense of Self, my intention for the New Moon in Sag is to establish financial security to use my knowledge to gain income and change or influence the lives of people around me.

I want to be a great mother to Messiah and right now that means being courageous enough to stand up to doctors, family, and friends who may try to make their views and beliefs my own.

I want to be my own version of a "mother" and not what my mother is or what Jackson's mom is.

My intention is to always manifest a life of abundance.

I pray for abundance in food, healthy for Messiah and I, and an overall better lifestyle.

NMRK

December 15, 2016

It was around this time last year that Messiah was conceived–
My greatest creation.

This year, I plan on creating my book, Like Water For Chocolate City.
I am closer to finishing and am putting all energy light and guidance
from the universe into it. I am creating products to sell through I AM
MELANIN and I'm continuing Melanin Book Club. I am creating for
myself and Messiah.

I am a mommy. I now have to balance women and children's interests
which is what I've always wanted to do.

As I am thinking and acting toward becoming a doula, I am thinking
about going to midwifery school. Jackson says it's good to have options/
back up plans, but I guess I never needed them, I just always figured it
must not have been meant to be.

But he's right.
We have to have back up plans, options, avenues, and different streams
of income. We're all not just good at one thing.

2017 will be the year of creative expression.
2017 is for my art.
My golden year.

December 19, 2016

Hey Mama's Baby,

You are currently sitting in a rocker, staring right at me with the biggest eyes, blowing spit bubbles. I decided to take some time to catch you up on all that's been going on. My maternity leave ended two weeks ago so I've been bringing you to work with me these last couple days. It hasn't been too much of a hassle but the weather is starting to get cold, and more people, including me are getting sick or just getting over a cold. You are perfectly healthy, thankfully, and completely unvaccinated. I hope to keep it that way. You deserve it.

It has truly been a journey these last couple months since you entered the world. I've been sick more often than not but still breastfeeding you and keeping you close to me at all times. Everyone who has met you, fell completely in love with you at first sight. You are that beautiful. It's hard enough not staring at you all day.

You're energy has changed our lives so much and I'm just now starting to feel like "myself" again.

I want to thank you for saving me.

I don't know what path I was on before I found out I was pregnant. I suppose I was close to giving up on my dreams and not following through with my goals. Then along came Messiah and now I feel more determined than ever to make you proud and keep you happy. I even think that your happiness is more important than my own. I pray for your health and happiness everyday. I pray that I become a better person for you, with you. I pray that I embody everything that you need in a mom.

2 months Postpartum

January 7, 2017

It's taken me seven days into 2017 to sit down to reflect and write out some goals. And a plan for how I'd like to accomplish them.

January 14, 2017

Three months postpartum and after having my wisdom teeth and 2 baby teeth extracted (with no pain meds!) I am on the road to healing, fully. Hopefully this time with no pain! I'm chanting (soon) for that! My mouth is still numb and sore and, of course, irritating. I miss food.

As the Full Moon energy is fully engulfing me, I am manifesting Like Water for Chocolate City and financial wealth in 2017.

February 3, 2017

Goals for 2017:

Publish LW4CC
Build Melanin & Books
Build Cannabis Business

Full Moon | February 11, 2017

Gratitude:

To the ancestors and elders.
To the universe and the future of the race.
To my love, Jackson (who's love I should take time to put into words to fully expression my admiration) who redefines peace
And love, over and over.
My two best friends.
My family.

I only want what's best for us, as a whole. Everyday I chant for our happiness and for our financial abundance; for a house for us to grow. I no longer want to live pay check to pay check, worrying about eviction notices, paying all our money to bills.

We will have income to travel, to buy everything that we want. We will own a home. We will never have insecurities about food or shelter, ever.

This month of 2017, I want to manifest everything that my ancestors deserve. All financial wealth, abundance, and land.

2017 Focus + Consistency

- Birth Business: Doula \\ Prenatal + Postpartum
- Bookstore: Black Books & Culture
- Apothecary: Cannabis, Herbs, Tea, Soap

February 21, 2017

Everyday I fall more in love with Jackson and more in love with Messiah. My best friends. I love them so much.

When Kristina died, I thought I would never have another best friend, but Jackson came into my life and my heart has finally healed.

I love him so much.

February 11, 2017

Hey Mama's Baby,

Thank you for trusting me. For holding me. And for believing in me. I needed a cheerleader and you came along, kicking and screaming and crying and laughing and smiling and playing and loving and loving and loving. My beautiful, peaceful baby. I love you.

These last four months have been an amazing journey, one of many ups and downs. I battled for a long time after birthing you with severe head-aches. So severe, I ended up in the emergency room a few times. And you were right there with me. You and daddy. The two of you spent several hours in the car in the hospital parking lot waiting for me. And me, I was in the hallway of the hospital emergency room, laid out on some bed being given painkillers through an IV. In hospitals, you could always tell who was rich and who was poor by how quickly one receives care. The last time I was in there ER, I came in at four and left exactly at midnight. I don't feel poor. But I have no money and I'm currently on medicaid. We will rise up. These days will be distant by the time you understand this. These times will be long gone.

We are working hard. Daddy and I. Everything we want will manifest.

Today we took you to the new African American Museum of History and Culture. You were the perfect baby. You were observant and smart. You were great. Daddy and I have so much fun hanging out with you and teaching you new things. Last weekend we took you to your first movie at the theaters, *I Am Not Your Negro*, a documentary about James Baldwin. You really enjoyed it.

You also attended your first SGI District Discussion Meeting a couple weeks ago. You really love to hear us chanting, Peace Baby. I'm so proud of you. You are the perfect addition to mommy and daddy's tribe. Did I mention you and daddy are best friends and I can stare at you two all day? You bring me joy.

Love,
Mommy

March 12, 2017

It's 6:34am

Messiah is nursing and holding my journal open as I write.
He's also being curious about what I'm writing here.
"I love you so much," I told him, and kissed him.
And made him continue feeding.
He's still curious.

His big brown eyes opened at 5:45am and would not fade close again, so
I'm up writing and praying and getting in tune with time.

Messiah reminds me that time as we know it, is not in tune with our natural clocks. Everything about him is natural so I need to follow his lead.

He came to teach me.

March 25, 2017

Hey Mama's Baby.

I've been so grateful for being able to breastfeed you exclusively for over 5 months now. You're five months old and teething and fussy right now but it's adorable and I love you and you're brave and we're getting through it. I'm excited for you. It's spring time and you're growing! My little flower. I couldn't have pictured a more beautiful boy.

Today we were attempting to go to the cherry blossom festival in D.C. since the weather is the warmest it's been this year so far. Spring is definitely springing and I am hoping to continue to manifest all of the seeds of abundance that I have planted.

I am happy that you and daddy are becoming members of SGI. It is such a tremendous benefit and honor to me. You love chanting and I am so excited to see you grow in such fortune and peace in our household. This is what I have dreamed up for you.

Now it is time to act on my dreams to be open to receive all the gifts of abundance, wealth, good health, and prosperity that is due to us.

Hey Mama's Baby,

You are nursing in my lap as I type this letter, slowly falling into your evening nap. I love you. You sweet, hilarious, loving, silly, baby boy. You are my light. I am slowly starting to feel like myself, like the cloud of new motherhood is fading and I can finally see everything more clear. And everything is beautiful. I'm so happy. These last few months have been a rollercoaster but I've enjoyed the ride knowing that each day is an opportunity to start anew. One day at a time, little one.

So you're teething like crazy and you crawled for the first time three days ago! You've been enjoying eating your new foods: bananas, broccoli, oatmeal, pears, apples, sweet potatoes, and green beans. Your daddy gave you a bath for the first time by himself yesterday. He was nervous. It was funny for me. He's getting the hang of things. Be patient with him. Daddy is truly wonderful and I couldn't be more happy of the family we are growing into.

Daddy is working hard and I am too. We will be wealthy and smart and will teach you to do the same. We are growing with you. My little prince. My Buddha-head. I will be starting my doula training next month, which will be the start of my birthing business. I'm also focusing on gardening and cultivation of cannabis. I want to use my passions to travel and help you to experience things that I never thought I would. And daddy will be our pilot and we will go everywhere we want. You've given me focus and I am thankful for these last seven months and almost 27 years of life.

Wow. I am exactly where I wanted to be at almost-27. Happy. Healthy. And making love. I will be publishing my book by the end of the summer. I hope that it inspires people to overcome, to never giver up, and to move beyond the box society ties to force us in. To love in spite of. To trust the universe or what ever Gods may be. To trust the journey, and one day when you read these words I hope it will inspire you, too. To be bold and confident. To not just dream and plan, but to live out loud.

This month starts a new phase for me and for you too. I've reached gold;

This new moon I am using to manifest a life of financial wealth.

Through publishing my books and starting my business, I am using this energy to begin my new life. From this moon onward. I am the richest woman alive.

All peace and light my Little One,
I hope you'll enjoy our adventure.

August 4, 2017

Hey Mama's Baby,

You are 10 months old + 2 days. I love and appreciate this journey more and more everyday. Every morning I have the pleasure of waking up to your smiling face and right now, you are sleeping peacefully next to me as I write to you. You've grown so much since my last letter. You have two teeth, and three more coming in! You are a strong and handsome baby boy. You are so calm and so sweet, Messiah. I am so proud of the personality and sense of humor that you've already developed. You had a check up at the doctor yesterday and you are perfectly healthy, 15lbs and 28 inches. You love trying new foods and hanging out with daddy. Your first word was "the" and you won't stop saying dada all day long and of course daddy loves it.

We'll be visiting Chicago in two weeks. It will be your very first plane ride and it'll be the first time meeting my mom, your grandma and auntie and uncles. I'm sorry it took this long for you to meet my family. I suppose it is all a part of the story... The story of my family and the work that we have to do to heal our hearts. I'm healing my heart for you and for daddy. Every day is difficult but you constantly teach me to be gentle, and careful. I'll admit that I sometimes yearn for more carefree days, less structure, and less routine, that comes with motherhood. But I love this life. I wake up each day full of gratitude.

I am thankful.

Two months ago, you were 8 months old at the time, I attended my first doula workshop so that I will be able to support mamas who will be giving birth. You attended the workshop with me and was such a great baby the entire time! Everyone loves you Messiah. That's exactly what I want you to inspire in people, love and peace.

From this I hope to start my own business, and build, build, build, all for us and our people. I think learning how to birth babies is vitally important to our survival as a race, so I'm considering becoming a midwife. A Certified Professional Midwife. I'm building my doula business and fundraising for my non-profit Melanin & Books at the same time. I'm writing and working, and still spending all my days with you.

I'm plotting. I'm still very much learning as much about cannabis as I possibly can, for a future business of mine. Prosperity. Wealth. I promised myself I would never work for white people again, now look at me. Building my nation.

We'll be moving into a new place soon and I'm hoping we will be able to grow more as a family. You have so much to learn and so much to explore. Thank you for letting me document all of it.

I love you.

It Takes A Village: Messiah's Birth Story
November 2, 2017

Let's be real. Having a baby is a trip. Motherhood is a real journey. Giving birth is like being reborn and my journey into motherhood has very much been like navigating through these phases of growth sometimes rather simply, with ease and grace, and other times stumbling, or more literally, crying my way through. Motherhood can be completely overwhelming and then at other times there's the shear joy and gratitude that comes from being able to cuddle, kiss, nurse and love on this baby that I've created in love and carried for nearly the whole of 2016. Childbirth is a miracle.

As the ancient African proverb states, it takes a village to raise a child, and as I have learned more recently through my journey into motherhood it also takes a village to *birth* a child. As I hold my beautiful brown baby, I am reminded of truth and purity and all that I have chosen to endure for the health and well-being of my little boy– who is now 1 year old. He reminds me of love and honesty and the responsibility I have to share that with others, and to teach and mold future generations of black children.

Throughout my entire pregnancy with Messiah, I had heard horror stories from first-time moms of 15+ hours of labor, with unheard of amounts of pain, women needing all types of drugs for pain relief and stories of how birth is disgusting and unpleasant, how doctors and nurses are usually rude, demanding, and impatient during labor. I had rarely heard women talk about their actual labor positively, if they told stories of it at all. That is, until I started to seek out the narratives of women who enjoyed giving birth and viewed birth as a peaceful, loving, spiritual, (and orgasmic) experience.

Whether we experience some pain or no pain, childbirth is the most natural experience on earth. I had always dreamed of having a home birth and throughout my entire pregnancy I battled with the idea that in some ways I would have to relinquish control of my body and my baby to medical professionals who wouldn't know me or my vagina from the next woman and potentially birth in a place completely unknown and foreign to me. My pregnancy really made me realize this sort of unconscious distrust that I'd had in hospitals and doctors who often view pregnancy and birth as a surgical, unnatural procedure requiring all types of intervention. I knew that I would have to take control of my healthcare from the very beginning, through education, research, and my own intuition.

I felt completely empowered to own my pregnancy and my birth experience. As women, especially women of color, we often relinquish the power that we have over our bodies and pregnancies without even realizing that we're doing it. We easily submit to our doctor's opinions without doing our own research. We willingly accept the advice of other women and our family, no matter how outdated, disproven, or misinformed that advice may be. We are the experts of our bodies and our babies, whether we have a medical degree or not. Women have been birthing babies since the beginning of time and without the assistance of doctors for just as long. It's instinctual.

For me, owning my pregnancy meant maintaining a healthy, balanced diet, or because of nausea, sometimes not. Drinking gallons and gallons of alkaline water and herbal tea. Reading, researching, and doing prenatal yoga religiously. I rode my bike. I slept when I needed to. I cried when I wanted to. I was completely crazy and at times irrational but it was all a part of the process. I found a healthier alternative to drinking that sugary glucose drink that doctors try to make mamas drink to test for gestational diabetes. I switched doctors, multiple times, until I found the midwives and the birthing center that was right for me and my family. I even changed insurance providers. I resigned from my amazing but tiring gardening job cultivating medicinal marijuana and settled at a non-profit organization founded by Black women that offers maternity support to low-income moms and that would let me bring Messiah to work with me post-maternity leave. I found my village and child birthing classes that fit my lifestyle--which is sadly too often inaccessible to low-income, young, Black, first-time, not married but not single moms, like me.

I had the birth that I had been chanting, meditating, and praying for. I believe that all women are entitled to a positive, peaceful birth experience, whatever that means to her. "Women birth how they live," a midwife said to me when I was pregnant and for me it was completely

191

true. If my mother could have four children naturally, I knew without a doubt that I could too. Although I had planned to have a water birth, and was even a little disappointed that Messiah's birth didn't go exactly as I planned-- with my doula present, and pictures and videos to share, I am very grateful to have had an intimate moment at home with just the three of us and I am even more grateful that both Messiah and I are healthy and safe. But if so many women are giving birth in situations where they may feel they have no control, scared, uninformed or unsupported, what does that say about the lives of women in our society as a whole? I hope that we begin to change the way we view birth and pregnancy in our communities and take real ownership of our reproductive rights.

I gave birth to Messiah on October 2, 2016. Ten days before the doctor's guess date. It was a rainy Saturday and I had no idea that I was in labor. I had spent the morning organizing our nursery and meditation room, doing prenatal yoga, and listening to my Hypnobabies tracks. Hypnobabies is a childbirth course that uses hypnosis or hypo-birthing to help families have a peaceful and natural birth. After binge watching Luke Cage on Netflix, Jackson and I took a long nap. I made brownies while Jackson went out to get Chipotle for dinner. Baby cravings. Around this time, I had started feeling what I thought at the time were Braxton Hicks. They were barely noticeable and only caused a little discomfort, so I didn't take them for any serious labor contraction, or what Hypnobabies likes to call Pressure Waves.

After an hour or two, I had barely touched my Chipotle and was disgusted by the brownies that I had been craving just hours before. Jackson, my amazingly patient and peaceful fiancé, birth partner, and Messiah's daddy, read the hypnosis script to me in bed to help me relax, which had become our nightly routine while we were taking the birthing class. I realized that I had some spotting which I knew meant labor was coming either within a few hours or a couple days and as I started to become nervous, the script really helped to soothe me and prepared my mind for the experience that my body and my baby would soon have.

After we finished the script it was around 11pm. I had some more spotting so I finally decided to tell Jackson. "That's a good thing!" He said, "That means he's coming." His words instantly melted away all of my fear and hesitation. We thought that we'd have between several hours and a few days until labor would pick up because this was my first birth and there is this idea that first-time moms are usually in labor for several hours to a few days before any baby arrives; we didn't worry. We had planned to have a water birth at a birthing center with midwifes and our doula supporting us. Since Messiah's bags were already packed we just had to get our things ready. Nonetheless, we starting packing our birthing bags to prepare for the birthing center as the whole idea of actually having a baby started to seem more real.

Before I could even put my things in my bag, my Pressure Waves (a.k.a contractions) became more intense and uncomfortable. I wouldn't describe it as pain, more like heavy pressure in my pelvis, making it uncomfortable for me to walk or move too quickly. I immediately think to take a bath to help ease the discomfort, so I take a quick bath. The pressure waves were coming more regularly now so Jackson calls the midwife who tells us to start to time them and call her back in 45 minutes. I get out of the bathtub and we go to the couch to start to time the contractions. It's 12:45am at this point, and the waves are now around 3-5 minutes apart and move from 30 seconds to almost 2 minutes in duration. I had the intense urge to push so I did, and after three of those, I gave birth to Messiah Maxwell around 1am. Right there, on the couch in our living room. With a Hypnobabies track playing on my phone, I sat there, in between Jackson's legs, on the black leather sectional and birthed our baby. "His head is coming out," I remember saying so calmly like I knew what was going on the whole time. I didn't. And definitely neither did Jackson. I had never seen him so frantic. Running for towels and stumbling on the phone with the midwife. It was classic.

Imagine our surprise.

Our accidental, unassisted home birth. It was the perfect birth for me. Really. Messiah came into the world perfectly healthy. 6 pounds, 7.5 ounces, and 20 inches of Black boy joy. If Messiah's birth story sounds perfect, magical, peaceful, and wonderful, it's because it was all of those things. Because Messiah himself is all of those things and because our bodies our perfectly capable of birthing without intervention. For that I am very proud. Literally, the moment we got off the couch, is when the real journey began.

Motherhood

February 13, 2018

Hey Mama's Baby,

I thought I'd take the time to write this letter to you while you're down for your afternoon nap. We've accomplished so much in the last 16 months and I'm so proud to be your mom. You started walking at 15 months which, doesn't seem that long ago especially considering how well you get around now. We also stopped nursing at 14 months, which I still kind of miss.

You are a curious little boy, and guess what, you love books like mommy. We took our first trip to the library and got your first library card last week. It was an adventure. Your favorite book, is my favorite children's book, *Whistle for Willie*. You can talk pretty well too! Mama, dada, hi, hello, bye bye, apple, happy, open...are only some of the words you know and say well. You've learned so much in such a short time. And I have to!

I completed my doula training, childbirth educator training, and completed certifications in herbal remedies and cannabis. You've been my motivation this whole time, so thank you. One day we will have a better life than the one that we have now and you're the reason. One day I will be a published writer and midwife, traveling and telling the stories that need to be told. And you? You are going to be a great big brother.

Mommy is currently 28-29 weeks pregnant with your little brother or sister, who is kicking as I type this. Motherhood has challenged me in so many ways; but it has for certain made me a better person and I'm also sure that if I wasn't a mother right now, I'd be empty. You light up my whole world with your smile. You fill my heart completely with your kisses. I am a servant to you. You are a God, Messiah and your sibling too.

Thank you for saving me.

I will spend the rest of my life praising you, teaching you, loving you and protecting you. I can't promise that the sun will always be out and that we'll never have gray days but I promise to always keep you warm. I promise to never hurt you or break you or treat you less than a God.

The world we live in is lucky to have you here, you don't deserve this place. So I promise today to show you more. I hope in your lifetime you see the beauty that resides here on earth and I hope that I can share that with you. I have yet to see everything or learn everything so be patient with me.

It is just the beginning.

We have many worlds to travel.

Postpartum Reflection:
Navigating New Motherhood
February 4, 2018

I've decided that I both needed and wanted to reflect on my postpartum experience and my first year as a new mom. I am currently 26-ish weeks pregnant with Baby #2 and a happy healthy 15-month-old baby toddling around after me. I was surely surprised when I found out that I was pregnant again, somewhere around the time Messiah was 11months old. I was mostly surprised because I was still breastfeeding at the time and as I was told then, breastfeeding is a good form of birth control postpartum (which is kind of true but only up until around 6 weeks). Anyway, still feeling empowered by my accidental unassisted homebirth with Messiah and the power of pregnancy and motherhood in general, I was overjoyed by the news. Within the last few weeks, however, I realized that I needed to be more intentional with my postpartum support and recovery in ways that I failed to do as a first-time mom. One way that I'm doing that is by honestly reflecting and healing from my last experience. (*The Cannabis Doula advice: Expectant moms, please create a postpartum plan and back-up plan to go with your birth plan!*)

My thrust into motherhood has been filled with many challenges that I was ill-prepared for during my postpartum period. I had spent so much time during my first pregnancy planning the perfect birth (that didn't even go as planned) and little to no time or thought went to what will actually happen when the baby gets home and the help I'll need recovering from childbirth. Motherhood, and pregnancy in general, I've found, is so much of a mystery until you actually experience it and its symptoms. This is only the case because of how individualistic our society has become. Where we should be gathering as women and celebrating certain Rites of Passages like getting our periods, learning how to heal our bodies and wombs with herbs, and the passing down of rituals, like postpartum healing methods, we simply don't anymore. Is giving birth in our community an experience that we'd just rather not talk about? I really hope to change that, especially in my family.

My (first) postpartum experience started like this:

Immediately after giving birth to Messiah, we called the midwife back and she directed us to call the ambulance to be transported to the hospital. I had never even entertained the idea of going to the hospital to give birth, so I was not prepared for the hospital protocol surrounding labor and delivery. I didn't even know which hospitals were in the area or anything about their maternity outcomes. Being rushed to the hospital on a stretcher after having already given birth was nothing short of ridiculous. Even after telling the paramedics, who informed the hospital that we were coming, that both Messiah and I were fine and that this was not an emergency, no complications, we were still treated as such.

When we got to the hospital, the paramedics wheeled us into labor and delivery where the nurses just sat there looking at us. Literally, shocked I guess at the fact that I was holding my newborn in my arms. They didn't know what to do or make of the situation. The paramedics had to explain to them that we had just called and that we had the baby at home and that we were okay. They go into full panic mode, make Jackson fill out a bunch of paperwork and take Messiah and me into a private room. There had to be like five nurses and two OBs in the room, all talking and asking me questions at the same time. They say that they need to hurry up and cut the umbilical cord, I tell them that we are delaying the cord clamping, they push until I give in by saying that the cord had already stopped pulsing. We had planned for Jackson to cut the cord, but he was separated from us in that moment which felt like forever. The fact that we were met with such panic and chaos is still so unbelievable to me considering how empty, quiet, and bored the staff seemed to be as we arrived. I decline most of the newborn interventions (bathing, vitamin K, eye drops, and vaccines), they put Messiah under the warmer by this time Jackson is in the room and I instruct him to go over to Messiah who had started to cry from being separated from me. The nurses continue to push to get me to allow them to do their newborn procedure. I sternly decline again, and again. By this time I feel my uterus beginning to contract to birth my placenta as the nurses continue to ask a million questions about my pregnancy and prenatal care. The resident OB in the room started to explain that she was going to give me Pitocin and that they had to start an IV. I decline. "Do you even know what Pitocin is for?" She responded in the most condescending tone. I explained to her what it is and what its for. My answer wasn't thorough enough for her so she then starts to scare me into letting her give me Pitocin by saying that if I don't get Pitocin I will risk bleeding out and hemorrhaging to death. "I'll take the risk," I told her declining again. I really wasn't being an asshole. I was confident in what I knew and confident that both my baby and I were healthy and fine without any unnecessary interventions. After birthing my placenta, I tell them that I was planning to keep my placenta. They tell me that in order for me to do that I would have to remove the placenta from hospital grounds within an hour or they'd have to keep it. Thankfully, I was able to do that. I remember thinking at that moment, what the hell type of hospital is this?

The OB then explains that I had 3rd degree lacerations from giving birth and that I would need stitches. They try to give me Oxycontin for the pain, I declined–because I was exclusively breastfeeding and knew the risk that narcotics could present. They did not inform me that narcotics could potentially interfere with breastfeeding and I wonder what would have happened if I didn't do prior research. The OB is irritated with me at this point and her attitude is obvious. She stitches me up, rather aggressively, only giving me Lidocaine which is a topical pain reliever used as a numbing agent. I felt all of her pulling and tugging, for a tear that she said was not even a centimeter long, but since it was deep she felt it would not recover properly without them. She said it wouldn't even take twenty minutes. It felt like much longer and halfway through the process, she leaves to get and the male Attending OB who then directs her the rest of the way.

At this point I'm over it. I'd had such a beautiful birthing now I'm in a hospital where I had ended up spending my first two days postpartum, the first two days of being a mom. I couldn't even imagine going home as painful as it was for me to walk or try to use the bathroom on my own, because of the tightness of the stitches and the hemorrhoids I developed from my precipitous birth. The next few days are filled with nasty hospital food and nurses coming in every two hours making it impossible to get sleep or do anything and making me all the more uncomfortable. I was so emotional and vulnerable at that time, realizing that I had actually given birth to a real baby and that my mom and family had missed the whole thing. The rest of my hospital stay consisted of Jackson, Messiah, and I trying to get some rest and steadily being intruded upon by various hospital officials who wanted to draw more blood, run random tests, and vaccinate Messiah or poke and prod him with various things and when we declined they used persuasion and coercion to get us to agree to whatever they wanted. We weren't budging. I was so happy to leave that place and at the same time happy to have had some care for those two days.

We came home to peace and quiet. I was so thankful. Especially for Jackson, who had made various trips back home to get whatever I needed at the hospital and to clean up and make sure that everything was in place for Messiah's homecoming. We both knew, especially after leaving the hospital, that we didn't want company while we got adjusted to our new life as a family of three. The next day, Jackson had to return to work, and I'd be at home alone with Messiah. I was still in a manageable amount of pain but it took almost a week or two to walk normally, without pain and discomfort as the too tight stitches dissolved. Not to mention the early discomfort from nursing and cluster feeding literally every hour. On top of caring for my newborn and myself, showering and preparing meals, I also had to consider any cleaning I'd need done. It was a lot and I had some help, thankfully, but not nearly as much as I had planned for or even thought I'd need.

I had my placenta encapsulated which helped tremendously with my mood and energy. However, not long after giving birth I started to have really bad headaches. They'd come on randomly and would be intensely painful. Follow up appointments with my midwife only left me with pain killers that were either safe for breastfeeding or that required me to take them in between nursing sessions. Still the headaches persisted and I ended up in the emergency room two times and urgent care a few times as well because the pain was so brutal. I had no idea what was going on. Doctors ran blood work and I had CT scans that revealed nothing as to why I was having such terrible headaches. I'd use acupressure and any other natural method to try to relieve them and it worked for a while but persisted until Messiah was around four months old. Then one day I thought that maybe I had an impacted wisdom tooth that could be causing these headaches. I did some research and went to see a dentist, who confirmed that I had several teeth that needed to be removed.

If you think childbirth is painful, you've never had six teeth (four wisdom teeth and two baby teeth) pulled in one day with only Novocaine during the operation and mild pain relievers afterwards. I endured a lot of pain all so that I could continue to nurse Messiah with no interruptions. I was in pain for weeks following the surgery and have yet to fully recover due to slight nerve damage. My postpartum period started off pretty rough. I returned to work three months postpartum and was able to bring Messiah to work with me, which was all love but still very challenging in its own ways. I was able to be amongst other Black moms who were nursing their children so I thankfully experienced little isolation during that time. Postpartum depression is another thing. I've definitely had my rollercoaster ride of balancing emotions, facing baby blues, and dealing with depression because of all of this. It's an ongoing thing that I constantly have to check for. Whether it was from not feeling supported, being extremely exhausted and sleep deprived, or experiencing discomfort from those headaches and toothaches, I struggled with depression in my early postpartum days, as most moms do.

I would have loved for my mom and sister and close girlfriends to have been close enough to support me following the birth of my baby, but it just didn't happen that way. New motherhood can be extremely isolating and for various reasons. Having to adapt to a whole new life of being careful, as opposed to my usual carefree lifestyle, putting my baby before anyone or anything (sometimes myself), and the idea that we aren't supposed to ask for help as a new mom is stressful, intimidating, and unfortunately driven by the culture we live in. So with this baby I'm hoping to do things a bit differently. I'm focusing on not only preparing for a healthy, easy birth but also for a much lighter postpartum experience. I'm centering my self-care and making sure that I'm eating well, resting, and taking time to heal which will include belly binding, herbal baths and teas, and other postpartum rituals. I'm also considering getting a postpartum doula, if the support of family falls through again, instead of carrying the load on my own shoulders and not realizing that I need support. It takes a village to raise a child, and to birth a child–so that mama can get some sleep! I'll need all the sleep and support I can get with a toddler and a newborn!

The Cannabis Doula advice: Mama, don't be afraid to ask for help! No matter how you feel, it won't make you a bad mom. Plus, no one should be coming over to see the new baby if they aren't bringing you something or helping you in some way!

Peace & Love.

Making Informed Decisions
in Pregnancy & Childbirth
March 3, 2018

I recently made it past my 28th week of pregnancy! I realized that even as a doula and childbirth educator giving birth to my second child, it is still especially important to know and understand all of the choices and options that are available to me in the care of my pregnancy simply because I am a young Black woman and we are so often taken advantage of when it's time to make these important, sometimes life or death, decisions.

This pregnancy has been as much of a challenge as my first pregnancy in understanding my health insurance policy and navigating the tiring process of choosing care providers. In a perfect world, I would have kept the same midwives from the birthing center I had planned to give birth at a little over a year ago but it didn't work out as easily. I had recently moved to another city/state, over an hour away in traffic, and commuting that far to make prenatal appointments and to make it there in time to give birth was too much of a hassle. I also wasn't truly satisfied with the care I was receiving and because I didn't give birth there last time, I had no real desire to continue care with that specific practice. After doing a bunch of research and making numerous calls, I decided to switch to another birthing center where I've been receiving care for the last couple of weeks and in doing that I also ended up switching insurance providers. It was a process but I'm so confident that I made the right decisions. We are receiving much more personalized care in a smaller, more comfortable setting closer to home. Plus, my health insurance overall is much better.

These are important decisions to make during or before pregnancy. Your care provider, (whether you choose OB-GYNS, Nurse-Midwives, or Homebirth Midwives to administer your care) can ultimately determine the quality of your care–in other words, their practice and beliefs will be a factor in your birth experience and outcome. Choose your care providers wisely. Not all physicians or midwives view birth as a natural, spiritual experience some view it as a medical procedure that requires drugs and surgery. Some hospitals treat birth as an emergency requiring constant monitoring and intervention. Likewise, not all insurance companies place maternal and child care as a priority. It is very important to research providers, hospitals, birth centers, and know your health coverage and with all of that information make an informed decision on your care. Even if, like me, you just gave birth within the last year or two—childbirth education must be ongoing.

Making informed decisions also extends to options in testing and other medical interventions during pregnancy as well as newborn interventions such as vaccines, and other medical decisions that you may encounter. I recently asked my midwife for an alternative to having to drink the glucose drink. We all know the dreadful glucose drink that I, personally, want nothing to do with. Usually at the 28th week of pregnancy, expectant mothers are often required to do a glucose screening to test for gestational diabetes. Gestational diabetes can be very serious, causing high blood sugar, affecting the health of both mom and baby. There are few symptoms associated with gestational diabetes and it is only diagnosed through blood work. It can lead to preeclampsia (toxemia) and depression often resulting in cesarean birth. It's serious, and a lot of providers will take testing for it very seriously as well. A sugary 50g glucose drink is usually given to the mom to drink then after an hour your blood is drawn and the amount of sugar in your blood is assessed to see how efficiently your body processes the sugar. I've heard so many women talk about how disgusting this drink is, how sweet it is, how it can make you nauseous, etc. but rarely do we discuss what is in this glucose drink and the alternatives to drinking it.

There are options and it's important to know them because your provider will usually do what is considered the norm without explaining alternatives and risks. I had to drink 8oz. of grape juice and eat 1/2 of a banana. Literally that's it. My midwife explained that the glucose drink gives a more accurate result but both options have the same amount of sugar for your body to process. Some moms may not have an issue with drinking glucose or may feel it is medically necessary for them and their baby and that's fine too!

What's important is that you made an informed decision in YOUR care.

Use your B.R.A.I.N.

Make informed decisions for your medical care (or for any really important decision:

B (Benefits):
What are the benefits to you and/or baby?

R (Risks):
What are the risks to you and baby?

A (Alternatives):
What other options are available?

I (Intuition):
What does your intuition tell you?
How does the decision make you feel?

N (Necessary/Not Now):
What happens if you do nothing?
Is it necessary?

Take the appropriate time to discuss your options with your provider and birth partner—with most decisions you will have time to research and discuss before having to make a final decision.

The goal is not necessarily a zero-risk choice, but the choice with the most acceptable risk for *you*.

Yoga & Chiropractic Care During Pregnancy
March 28, 2018

Exercise is very important for a healthy pregnancy and an easier child-birth. Getting up, being active, and moving around not only helps to open up the hips and pelvis, it also helps during labor to ease the discomforts that may come with contractions. Yoga has been my exercise of choice for both pregnancies and I especially enjoy yoga because it helps me to increase my flexibility, concentration, and breathing which can all help while giving birth. Yoga also helps with my occasional insomnia (a good yoga practice can really wear me out!) and it helped with the soreness and ongoing pain in my tailbone, which up until recently I thought was just a part of pregnancy.

I struggled (and wobbled about) when I was pregnant with Messiah and even afterwards, and the occasional pain in my tailbone has continued throughout this pregnancy as well. Now, running behind a toddler and maintaining a weekly yoga routine while carrying the extra weight from this pregnancy (I've gained 25lbs so far) has proved too much for my poor sacrum. If you've ever been walking around the grocery store, or bending over to pick something up, or even just getting off the couch and that sharp pain shoots up your ass then you know exactly what I'm talking about. I've been spending the last week or two getting comfortable with my heating pad AND I finally went to see a chiropractor.

Not only am I seeing my chiropractor twice a week (she is phenomenal and very gentle with me and baby), I'm also wondering why didn't I do this sooner and why isn't chiropractic care part of my prenatal care?!

On most days I feel a lot better after getting adjusted, doing exercises, and getting some massage work. Chiropractic care is recommended during pregnancy, my midwife encouraged it, and it has tremendous benefits. It helps with my pain, obviously, but it also helps with my mood, sleep, and overall comfort in my pregnant body. Our bodies go through so much of a change when we are pregnant sometimes we need more support in getting adjusted than we realize.

I'll be seeing my chiropractor after I give birth as well and I can't wait to see how much lighter and more in tune I feel. Until I get my ass together (literally) I'll be taking it easy on the yoga and focusing more on walking and opening my pelvis. I have no problems taking it easy and focusing on getting rest as I near the end of my pregnancy.

I would love to hear how you mamas are staying fit and active during pregnancy and any experience you've had with chiropractic care to treat pregnancy related pain.

Giving birth is like running a marathon, we have to exercise during pregnancy to prepare for the workout body has to undergo to have a natural, healthy birthing and a happy baby.

On National Black Maternal Health Week | Why I Became A Doula
April 19, 2018

The First National Black Maternal Health Week (April 11th-17th) just ended and it brought up a lot of important statistics to share in regards to the state of Black women's health in the U.S. and allowed me to deeply reflect on my own life and experiences.

To put it simply, Black women are 3 to 5 times more likely to die in pregnancy, childbirth, or postpartum than our white counterparts and our babies are 2 times more likely to die in infancy than white babies. Mind you, these stats are worse depending on your city and hospital. To really put it in perspective about how bad these statistics are, you really have to consider a few important points. Black women in America are more likely to die of pregnancy related complications regardless of socioeconomic status and education level. In fact, Black maternal mortality is worse now than it was in the 1850s during slavery and it has gotten worse since my mom was having children over 25 years ago. Black women in the United States, one of the wealthiest countries in the world, are 243% more likely to die due to pregnancy/childbirth complications than white women. It is a harsh reality and it is an even worse reality for pregnant Black women who may be unaware of the racial injustices that are present in the health care system.

Last week, I was asked what inspired me to become a doula. While my background in Family & Child Studies and Family Social Services has led me to the work I do now, for me being a doula, a birthworker, and Black mother is a revolutionary act. This is how I've taken the injustice and harm being done to Black women and Black children on an everyday basis and found healing. This is how I use my voice and education to teach and heal the other Black women. To amplify and center our experiences, our opinions, and potentially impact our birthing outcomes.

I was inspired to be a doula by a very fierce mama that I met at a rally in Chicago, protesting budget cuts in childcare by the governor. A decision that would grossly and disproportionately affect Black women and children. She was a manager of a Black homeschool collective on the south side, one that I would go on to work at and learn so much from. She was married and mother of two little boys. She was also in seminary school with a very radical view of religious responsibility and very actively and radically involved in protests and social justice activism around the city. She became pregnant and gave birth to her third son only a few months before I birthed my first son. She offered advice and encouragement and insisted I get a doula, by letting me know how vital they are. We talked about raising our boys to be well-mannered and gentle men and the importance of that responsibility as Black mothers.

She will never know the impact that she had on my life, at a time when I was seeking the genuine sisterhood of Black women, especially older women, in my life. Watching her mother her boys, and other children in her care, was as profound as it was lovely. She passed away only eight months after giving birth to her third son due to pregnancy related complications. Everyday I do this work with her in mind. I do this work for the women in my family who have died postpartum, who have been pillars in maternal and child health, for my great-grandmother who was a midwife back when Black women weren't even allowed to birth in hospitals. For my closest girlfriends who have died during their childbearing years because their mental and physical health were ignored. They've empowered me in this journey.

I knew the statistics. These are more than just numbers for me, they are mamas that I've known, friends that have struggled through pregnancy because of inadequate prenatal care, childbirth education, and postpartum support. Doulas support birthing women emotionally, mentally, and physically during pregnancy and childbirth, and after. We provide childbirth education and breastfeeding support. We mother the mother at a very vulnerable time in her life. For Black women, having a doula for support during pregnancy and childbirth can literally be a matter of life or death. To have another Black woman, who has experience in providing family support and education, who can help educate and advocate for her is absolutely vital in navigating this health care system that is rooted in harming the bodies of Black women.

Very few people know or care to acknowledge that modern obstetrics and gynecology began by experimenting on the bodies of enslaved

Black women, with no anesthesia, and that birth control began as a means to control Black women's fertility and live births. It is believed by some doctors and even written in medical textbooks to this day, that Black women and infants experience less pain than others, are innately susceptible to illness, and this great maternal health disparity is due to our own imperfections and behaviors—statements that hold no validity and are absolutely rooted in racism.

It is important for Black women to know what we are up against from the moment we get pregnant in order to make the best choices for lives and for the health and happiness of our babies and families.

I want to thank the Black women who have been on the front lines of this revolutionary work, the Black midwives who have been outlawed from practicing on a professional level only to have hippy white women claim their traditional practices as their own, for all the women who have died in order for us to recognize this week and the importance of our maternal health. Thank you.

& I hope that with every client that I support, every class that I teach, and every baby that I give birth to, you may find honor and love in my work.

Mars' Earth Day Birthday
May 22, 2018

One month ago today, I gave birth to my second baby boy, Mars. I woke up around 4:30am on April 22nd, a Sunday morning, thinking I just had to use the bathroom. I had become so accustomed to the late night trips to the bathroom that often interrupted my sleep but I knew that baby would be coming any day, as I was nearing my 39th week of pregnancy. After using the bathroom, I started to feel pressure and knew that it may be time to go to the birthing center. I immediately felt a burst of energy, excitement, and a little bit of anxiety. Finally! Our main concern was making it to the birth center in time, since we had almost a forty-minute drive, and I had a history of birthing really fast. I was also concerned about making sure Messiah was cared for and not afraid during the whole experience. I had a list posted on the refrigerator of all the things I needed to grab and things I needed to do when I realized it was my birthing time. So I woke Jackson up and immediately went to my list and started gathering our birthing bags and getting Messiah's things ready.

As my pressure waves (contractions) began to feel more intense, I called the midwife, who told us to come right in. I started to feel like we wouldn't make it there in time. The midwife's voice on the phone was very reassuring in that moment and that helped me to release any fear I had around getting to the birth center. Because I was seeing the midwives in rotation I had no idea who would be on call to help birth my baby, and towards the end of my pregnancy I began to feel anxiety about possibly not having a Black midwife for various reasons. So hearing the voice of the Black midwife that I had been most comfortable with during my prenatal appointments, was very reassuring and affirming. I felt safe, and ready to bring my baby into the world.

We get everything together, get Messiah up, dressed and ready and Jackson loads the car. As we are leaving out of the door, I had a pressure wave that let me know that baby was coming very, very soon. I grabbed my laptop with my Hypnobabies tracks and immediately put my headphones in my ears. My pressure waves were intense every seven minutes for fifteen seconds the entire ride there. I felt my body preparing to give birth and the birth affirmations that I was listening to helped to prepare me mentally and also helped me keep the baby in until we made it to our destination. I had to be sure not scare Messiah by appearing to be in pain or distress but sitting upright, restrained by the seatbelt was not an ideal position to be in. I breathed through each contraction, not relaxing too much because I knew if I let go completely, I would have most certainly had the baby. I was doing my best to hold the baby in!

"Take your time," I'd say to Mars repeatedly with each pressure wave. With the really intense ones, Jackson would say "peace," reminding me to relax, placing his hand on my forehead or shoulder, like we practiced in Hypnobabies, he'd remind me to use my hypno-anesthesia. We pretty much flew to the birth center, which was thankfully how fast Jackson got us there.

We pull up to the parking lot and the midwife greets me at the car. She tells Jackson to grab Messiah out of the car and come right in, just in case I give birth soon–she didn't want him to miss it by unloading the car. As we walk inside I have a pressure wave, once we make it to the room I'd be birthing in I start to play my relaxation music. I immediately feel relaxed and peaceful. I make my way to the bed and ask the midwife if I can get in the tub, she says of course and has Jackson go fill the tub as she helps me get comfortable. In that exact moment I start feeling intense pressure and the urge to push. My water breaks and the midwife calls for Jackson to come back in the room. Messiah cries briefly as I'm in the bed on all fours with Mars' head crowning. The midwife helps guide my pushing to make sure I didn't have any tearing. I allowed my body to naturally push without trying to bear down or strain too much. "Reach down, grab your baby," my midwife says, helping to unwrap the cord from around his neck, "it's a boy!" I announce, overjoyed. Mars Osiris was born at 5:56am, 6lbs. 5oz. 20inches of Black boy beauty. Just ten minutes after making it to the birth center, and an hour & eleven minutes after my birthing time began.

Shortly after birthing my placenta, my doula arrives and Jackson and Messiah leave to get breakfast for all of us while Mars and I get breastfeeding and bonding initiated. There was a feeling of such love and peace that I had felt for everything going so smoothly...I enjoyed giving birth to Mars, and Messiah was so happy as well. He smiled and clapped when he saw that mommy gave birth to his little brother, "you did such a good job, Messiah! This is your little brother," we told him. Waiting for birth to reveal Mars' gender was the most amazing feeling for me–Jackson claimed to have known the whole time that it was a boy, so he wasn't at all surprised to find out.

In fact, Jackson was so calm, peaceful, and patient the entire morning which we had a good laugh about considering he had been up really late the night before watching a boxing match, drinking, and for the past few nights, falling for the same prank of me pretending that my birthing time was starting. I have such sincere gratitude for him, the best birth partner!

Jackson came back with breakfast and our family had arrived to help with Messiah. Soon after, Jackson cut Mars' umbilical cord and I showered while they did skin-to-skin. Once Messiah ate breakfast and left with family, Jackson and I ate as well and by noon prepared to go home with our newborn. What a perfect way to end the morning with our Earth Day baby in our arms, and in my arms he has been ever since.

Happy 1-month, Mars!

Happy Black Breastfeeding Week 2018:
Tips for Establishing Breastfeeding!
August 30, 2018

Breastfeeding is the best way to help birthing people recover after childbirth, learn mothering instincts, and initiate bonding and attachment with baby. It's also nature's way of ensuring that our babies are properly nourished, protected from illness and disease, and allowed to develop optimally. The American Academy of Pediatrics (AAP) recommends that babies be exclusively breastfed (no water, juice, formula, other fluids, or solids) for six months and continue breastfeeding until at least two years. Here are some ways you can get your breastfeeding relationship off to a good start with your little one:

Before your birth:
- Always keep in mind that your body knows exactly how to breastfeed your baby! Incorporate practices in your birth plan that support breastfeeding.
- Talk to women in your family or friends who are breastfeeding or have breastfed their babies. Learn about your family's history with breastfeeding.
- Join a support group of other nursing families.
- Consult with a Lactation Consultant or breastfeeding educator.
- Check out books on breastfeeding.

In the first hours after birth:
- Skin-to-skin immediately after giving birth encourages babies to nurse.
- Nursing during the Golden Hour helps the uterus to contract, birth the placenta, and provides nutrient-rich colostrum to the newborn.
- Delay newborn tests and other routine procedures until after breastfeeding has been established.
- Be patient with yourself and your baby as you both are learning to breastfeed.

In the first few days:
- Consider co-sleeping in the early days to help with late night feedings.

- Carry your baby! Wear your baby in a carrier to provide comfort and easier access to milk when it's time for baby to nurse.
- Ensure that baby is swallowing as they suckle and check for adequate wet diapers to make sure baby is nursing well.
- Make sure baby has a nice deep latch, and you both are in a comfortable position.
- Hold off on bottles and pacifiers for a few weeks to prevent nipple confusion.
- Pain medication used during childbirth, circumcision and other painful newborn procedures can interfere with an infant's ability to breastfeed.
- Never mix infant formula and breast milk together. If you must be separated from your nursling, pump and store your breast milk.

In the first few weeks:
- Build trust with your baby by responding to feeding cues.
- Be confident in your journey, no matter how challenging.
- If you have breastfeeding problems or if you're concerned about whether your baby is getting enough milk, contact a certified lactation consultant.
- Remember that breast milk is all the nutrition your baby needs for the first six months, and is recommended for the first two years!

If you have issues nursing:
If challenges arise and you are unable to breastfeed, encourage other ways to bond with your baby.
- Bed share or sleep in the same room with your baby.
- Wear your baby traditionally, or in a baby carrier. Remember, babies cannot be spoiled.
- Observe your baby and respond to their needs before they cry.
- Use skin-to-skin, massages, and bath time routines to encourage closeness.

Postpartum Planning & Preparation
June 14, 2018

Usually when you are preparing to have a baby, we're told to make a birth plan. Birth plans are a great way to learn about different birthing options and important choices that have to be made during pregnancy. As a doula, I usually have my clients create a postpartum plan as well. Postpartum planning takes more preparation in order to be successful. There is so much to consider for after the birth, new moms especially, wouldn't know---I sure didn't! Here are some tips to properly plan for or consider once you bring your little one home.

1. Padsicles

Padsicles are heavenly after having a baby. They are frozen pads with essential oils or herbs and aloe vera. They are very simple to make and take very little time. To make my padsicles, I steeped a mix of seven different herbs, added some aloe vera, and poured the mixture on top of two really big pads, for immediately after birth, and two maxi pads. I wrapped the pads back up and put them in the freezer until it was my birthing time. After giving birth, the coolness of pads felt amazing. The herbs and aloe vera smelled so good and offered immediate comfort. Some traditional practitioners won't recommend anything cold immediately after birth, if your padsicle is cold or frozen, I recommend alternating hot and cold, by sitting on heated seats or a heating pad while wearing your padsicle.

2. Postpartum Basket

Weeks before birth, I prepared a postpartum basket to keep all of my postpartum healing items easily accessible. Included in my basket were lots of maxi pads, Tucks pads, hemorrhoid cream, nipple butter, and mesh undies. Postpartum baskets are an awesome reminder for moms to take care of yourself! As a first time mom, I had no clue of what to expect during the first few weeks after giving birth. I was so focused on getting all the items the baby would need, I didn't even have pads at home! The second time around, I was more than ready with my lovely postpartum basket. This also makes a great gift for a new mom.

3. Meal Prep

Please, do your soul a favor! Prep your meals for at least two weeks or coordinate with friends and family to help buy your groceries, bring you food, or have it delivered to your home. If you have little ones, make sure you prep their meal and have snacks ready for them as well. Having food on deck, your favorite drinks and snacks, not only saves time but can help minimize the stress of worrying about what to cook. I had my favorite energy drinks, fruit, and granola bars at my bedside so I didn't have to worry about getting up to get snacks while I was in bed breast-feeding right after giving birth.

4. Herbal Sitz Baths & postpartum wellness herbs

Herbal baths aid in healing postpartum and can be relaxing to both mom and baby. I used a special blend of herbs that are specifically used during the postpartum period to support vaginal healing, bleeding, inflammation, and uterine contractions. My herbal blend will be available for purchase, or you can craft your own blend of herbs!

5. Hire a Postpartum Doula

If you know you'll need extra help around the house and adjusting with your new baby, consider hiring a postpartum doula. They can provide education, assist with meal prep, household cleaning, and caring for the baby while mom gets rest.

6. Consume or Encapsulate your Placenta

Take your placenta with you! Your placenta can provide lots of nutrients, help hormone regulation, and provide energy to new moms. You can add it to your daily smoothie, or encapsulate it. Whatever works for you.

September 17, 2018

It's happening. I can feel it.

Autumn it making its way around the corner, though the thick humidity and summer heat may tell you otherwise. I know better. The season is changing. As are we. Time is passing. Months have turned into years. Sometimes I flashback to three years ago and I could cry, all over again. Three years ago, I was twenty five years old and at the lowest point in my life.

I had experienced so much heartache and so much death, I was risking my own life for what I thought would prove my worth as a young, Black woman in this country. I wanted to die in order to teach white people a lesson on humanity. I was willing to fight. To put my body on the line. I didn't care about anything else. I'm Black, and I was angry.
(Do you know what their ancestors did to ours, and the generational trauma?!)

But fuck it. It's not my job nor yours to teach white people their humanity. Way too many brilliant Black minds have gone to waste trying to turn a mirror to white people. A people who can so easily gentrify an entire community of color and then walk around like we are the ones out of place.

If Martin, Malcolm, (and Assata, and Mumia, and MOVE, and Marcus, And Mandela, and so on and so on) can so eloquently, so boldly, and so powerfully tell white people who they are and absolutely nothing changes– how could I, a little Black girl, from 79th street in the most violent city in America, think my life would somehow magically make white people sit back, in their gourmet kitchens and silk robes, and think, "damn, you know what– here's some reparations. I deserve this life, and so do you. Here's some land. And some money. You know what, here's some more money. How 'bout some more justice, and equality, no, you know what– here's some equity. And some more money and land."

We want a future for our children. And all I'm saying is, in the past we haven't gotten that by being peaceful, or by being angry. We have to strategize and organize. We have to learn to play their game, then beat them at it. Unlearn and relearn. Un-school. In all areas.

Everything we've been taught is backwards. We have to return to the source, which is nature, and heal. Be rooted. Create.

We are at war and losing soldiers everyday.
We need to raise strong armies.
We need to build power and wealth.

I give up the notion that fighting white supremacy and capitalism and imperialism looks like me being poor is fuck.

I am wealthy because I believe in the power of people.
Capital and access comes to those who use their voice to impact change in the world.

Since I've kept quiet,
I meditated,
I've healed.

A Love Letter to Mars

September 23, 2018

Dear Mars,

You are the most beautiful and loving baby I've ever met. Your smile melts my heart. I've truly fallen in love with you in these short five months earthside. You've made my life so full. Each time that I hold you, I am all the more certain that I am exactly where I should be. You are the confirmation. And Messiah is very happy to have a brother.

Just a tad jealous.

You've really taught me to live in the moment, to be present, to be kind. You're calm, always. You eat well and you sleep well. You're very content and very happy. Your birth was magical, as are you.

My earth day baby, thank you for coming for me.

I realized there is still some healing that needs to take place on my behalf. From the past. From my childhood. In order for me to be a better mother. I'm continuing on this healing journey by sharing some moments in my life that have been hard for me, so that you will learn from it--in any way you choose.

I hope you will learn a lesson on love, and heartbreak, and community, on justice, and violence...

three

Indigo, looks down at her phone to a message about Mumia, instantly remembering who she was and of her purpose, and the obligation she had to her people. The haze of pregnancy and postpartum finally clearing up after 9 months, post-baby number two, Mars. Who she held tightly in her arms, nursing to sleep. Messiah, just 2 years old, playing intently nearby his mama.

Brother Pete's message was a gentle nudge from the ancestors to remember, even though Indigo was expecting it any day now it partly caught her by surprise. Did he forget about me? She often thought.

"Probably," she concluded, and decided not to reply to the message. Instead she tended to her babies, cooking dinner, or running, loving, and singing after them. Days pass in this way. That beautiful way of waking up to the soft pokes of a baby's foot and then going to sleep to their kisses. Their needs met. The dreams of all four of them, a mommy, a daddy, and their babies, a melanated family, all satisfied for now. Each living their version of happiness.

Indigo realized that it had been five years since she had decided to move to D.C., where she learned who she was, met Jackson, fell in love, and it was love that brought her back to him. It was love that brought them back together, in truth and in friendship, it was love that started their family, giving birth to Messiah and Mars. Five years ago it was that Indigo decided to, in the only way she knew how, turn her poison into medicine. It was that decision that allowed her to be who she is. But Brother Pete's message caused a bit of a stir in her, because after all, she remembered. For her babies, and her new life, had only caused her desire for African liberation to intensify. Her commitment to the Black family, honoring the Black woman, educating Black children, and uplifting the Black man was a full time job, one she did everyday at home. She knew her place in the Revolution.

"Are you being reactionary or revolutionary?" Brother Pete had asked, one evening years prior, as Indigo sat on his couch exasperated, after recalling for him how she had been out protesting and rallying with other young Black folks. "You must be tired, and I bet your shoes are run down now too, huh?" He asked, but already knew the answer. "Now you're going to have to buy some new shoes, and probably from one of these white people or corporations that you're out protesting against in the first place. See, y'all so busy fighting battles while they are winning the war! You don't think we did that already? So y'all wouldn't have to? If protesting or rioting worked, don't you think we would have won a long time ago?" Indigo didn't understand his anger in the moment, in fact, she thought he'd be proud that they were picking up where his generation had left off.

Brother Pete, one of the last living members of the original Black Panther Party was very well-known and respected in DC, and Indigo sat before him bewildered by his stupidity. And he was also baffled by hers. He had seen far too often young Black revolutionaries die from acting with emotion rather than logic and she had known far too many elders who had dropped the ball. "But do you feel better now?" He asked, and hugged her. He, too, had been there and he knew that Indigo, her generation and thereafter, would go where he and his had not. So he taught her what he knew. Introducing her to everyone that he knew as one of the greatest young revolutionaries of her generation and the future leader of the Free World. "She's the one," he'd tell people, insisting she go with him to the Mayor Bower's inaugural ball for this very purpose, to meet all of the uppity Blacks with money, status, and clout.

He'd spend hours lecturing her on world history, biblical history, and Black history never spoken of, making sure to answer every question she had, and he in return would ask questions of her to make sure she wasn't the Feds, for one could never really know. They'd spend hours on the phone, pouring through website after website, and book after book. Learning. He taught her the importance of owning a business and creating art, which is of equal importance. He talked to her about the elders and about the youth. At times, Indigo, so in need of the mentorship of older Black men, would just sit at his feet listening intently, cooking small meals for the two of them or whoever else was visiting, and roll his weed. They smoked, recorded Indigo's poetry, listened to revolutionary music with no purpose other than to learn from one another. Indigo would silently dream of what it must have been like to have a granddad nearby or a loving father figure to ask questions of and to cry to. Brother Pete had served a very important role during Indigo's time in DC, she later told him. He had helped to prepare her to be a better woman to Jackson and mother to her boys.

Of course, she remembered.

The
Cannabis
Doula

January 17, 2019

I begin this space with gratitude
And light.
This is a space of healing
And restoration.

This is a space of self-forgiveness
And self-love.
I am a sacred woman.
I offer peace and love to my
Foremothers, my ancestors, and my divine feminine.

I pray that I am able to gather Black women
who are whole, sacred, and committed
to healing other Black women and girls.

I pray for *Revolutionary Motherhood*.

May we take back our right to birth + mother.

I pray for the wombs of all Black women.
I pray that I am able to use my voice to speak truth + love.

Release me of fear, insecurity, anger, and distractions.

I attract wealth, money, prosperity, land.
I deserve to live lavishly.
I deserve to live in luxury.
I deserve the finest, I will have the greatest.
I have everything I need to live my dream.

Books, Bud, & Black Love Podcast
Reading List

February - Black History Month
Little Man, Little Man- James Baldwin
A Good Cry - Nikki Giovanni

March - Women's History Month
Heart of a Woman- Maya Angelou
Sula- Toni Morrison

April
Children of Blood & Bone- Tomi Adeyemi
Killing the Black Body - Dorothy Roberts

May
The Alchemist - Paulo Coelho
Native Son - Richard Wright

June
Black Skin, White Masks - Frantz Fanon
Jambalaya - Luisah Teish

July
Not That Bad - Roxanne Guy
Kindred - Octavia Butler

August
Mama Day - Gloria Naylor
Rise Dream - Walter Mosley

September
Beloved by Toni Morrison
Post-Traumatic Slave Syndrome - Joy DeGruy

October
Another Country - James Baldwin
Killing Rage - bell hooks

November
The Spook Who Sat By The Door - Sam Greenlee

December
Zora Neale Hurston - Bearricon
The Prophet - Kahlil Gibran

Cannabis Strains

*CBD-Dominant marijuana
and hemp*

Shark Shock
Painkiller XL
Bubba Kush
Hawaiian Haze

*Broad Leaf Marijuana
Also known as indica*

Grease Monkey
Blue Cheese
Gelato Cake
Salmon River

Broad Leaf Dominant

LA Chocolat
Girl Scout Cookies
Jelly Breath
gSpot
Mai Tai

*Narrow Leaf Marijuana
Also known as sativa*

Sour Diesel
Acapulco Gold
Sunshine #4
Golden Strawberry
Durban Thai
Durbon Poison
24k Gold

2/14/19

Greetings Dr. Greene

I am a cannabis cultivator and processor in Maryland. I work collectively, along with other cannabis growers, processors, and entrepreneurs of color, through Diaspora Hemp & Wellness to educate communities on the benefits of medical cannabis, laws and legalization, and provide professional caregiver services to licensed medical cannabis patients.

With the historic announcement of the Maryland House Bill 698 and the 2014 Farm Bill, the Maryland Department of Agriculture has recently established the Maryland Industrial Hemp Pilot Program that enables individuals to partner with institutions of Higher Education in the state of Maryland to conduct research projects on Industrial Hemp. My team and I would like to use this opportunity to research hemp to grow, process, market, and sell for its innumerable medicinal benefits.

I am interested in partnering with a university to conduct research on growing hemp for the extraction of CBD to produce various medicinal, health, and wellness products. We are hoping to partner with an HBCU that has the greenhouse space necessary to accommodate our research with the hopes of creating hands-on research and development opportunities for Black students in Industrial Hemp/ Medical Cannabis in Maryland and we are especially interested in collaborating with the staff and students at Bowie State University at the Center for Natural Sciences, Mathematics, and Nursing.

If you'd be interested in potentially partnering with us, let's schedule a time to meet to discuss the program and how we can work together. I hope to hear from you.

All the best,
Melanie Julion

Greetings Joy,

I am writing this to inquire about my application to be a medical cannabis patient in Maryland. I originally submitted my MMCC Patient application last year in August of 2018. There has been issue after issue involving submitting my application since then (it is now March 2019). I believe I've submitted four times now. As someone who needs medication, I can no longer afford to wait. I struggle with PTSD, anxiety, and was recently diagnosed with thyroid cancer, all of which can be treated with medical cannabis.

Is there any way that I can come in and speak with anyone, to show documentation in person, to receive assistance as soon as possible? The pictures that I've submitted cannot get any clearer (I cannot afford an HD camera.) Is there an option to scan document or send them through the mail? There has to be something, as quality of camera should not be a barrier to access medication. Please advise. Is the issue my address, my sources for proof of address, or my background?

I am available to come in to show proof of everything, as soon as possible.

1st application- Resided in Baltimore, I was told the my proof of address was not sufficient. And that I could not wear a head covering (which is in fact discriminatory considering my head covering is worn for spiritual and religious reasons. And many women, in Maryland, wear religious head coverings.) August 2018. The proof of address I provided were from Maryland State Department and an insurance bill.

At that point, I was undecided on whether or not to resubmit my application. However, I was encouraged to keep trying and I needed access to medication.

2nd Application- Moved to Silver Spring, MD in November 2018. So, I retook the picture. I submitted my photo and two new pieces of mailing. A Pepco phone bill (utility) and a letter from Maryland Department of Education (state department). November 2018. Application returned for proof of address.

*3rd Application-*Then I submitted another Pepco bill, a letter from Health & Human Services, & a copy of my signed lease

4th Application- The last application that I sent contained a new Pepco bill, a letter from Maryland health connection, a new letter from Dept. Health & Human Services.

As I await my pending 4th application, as not only a patient, but an entrepreneur in the cannabis industry, I can only hope that my application will be approved and that it is not being rejected, constantly, due to my race.

I work within the cannabis industry providing cannabis education, support, and care, especially for the equity of Black communities and women. I was previously a licensed cultivator in DC. I am appalled at the Maryland Medical Cannabis Commission. Our state is falling grossly behind in providing equity and cannabis care in comparison to other States. Not only are Black cannabis entrepreneurs not being supported through small business loans/lending, or grants, we also don't have access to land, equipment, or cannabis licenses that cost thousands of dollars to even submit applications for. Black patients are being largely shut out.

If Black people are going to get ahead in this industry in this state, The Commission has to do more in getting Black patients signed up and getting entrepreneurs access to funding in the industry! This is institutionalized racism and injustice.

I will be graciously awaiting your feedback and reply. I can best be reached by email and phone.

Best,

Melanie Julion

Welcome to The Cannabis Doula

This is my revolution. I'm pulling my seat up to the table. I found out I was pregnant, for the first time, while cultivating medical cannabis for a Black-owned cultivation center in DC. I had to make a really tough decision. I didn't know how I would coexist as a Black woman in the cannabis industry and now, a young Black mom in this space. There was no way. The taboo was way too apparent. The stereotypes, the misinformation, the propaganda and the stigma is all too real in Black communities. For example, you'll likely find that "there isn't enough research done on the benefits or harm of cannabis during pregnancy" yet cannabis received official medical recognition as a childbirth aid in the U.S. in the 1850s.

Essentially, the hard labor of cultivation was causing me a lot of physical stress (lifting 5 gallon buckets of water all morning is not easy when you have morning sickness) and the grow environment wasn't safe. So I resigned from my job, after really feeling like I had no choice. I was pregnant and isolated in a male dominated industry with no way to support or advocate for myself and my needs as a pregnant person. I resigned from doing something I'd wanted to do for so long–GROW Cannabis!

From there, I was drawn to birthwork where I began to cultivate my love of birth and supporting mamas and babies. Having little support during my pregnancy, especially in the first five months while I was working at the cultivation center, I became empowered to advocate for myself and other expectant families. One thing I've noticed since starting this journey, is the shame present in mothers who do decide to use cannabis. And there is a lot of us. And a lot of shame.

Cannabis is the most used "illicit drug" by pregnant women. So, my question now became: why are we so ashamed? So many women, mothers, I've personally worked with and talked to use cannabis to treat all types of pregnancy concerns. From severe nausea, to pain relief, to postpartum depression! First, I had to do a lot of my own self-acceptance when it came to my own cannabis use. I do consume cannabis, medically and recreationally, and as a melanated woman, mama, birthworker, and cannabis entrepreneur, I stand by that.

I applaud all women who choose cannabis! So often Black moms get discouraged from seeking doula support for the fear they have of being judged for their consumption! In order do my best work as a doula, I think it is so important to bring my whole self to the table, so that I can truly advocate for us. I've been working tirelessly to combine my knowledge and experience in the cannabis industry and my work as a doula. I recently realized I've been educating pregnant people about cannabis this whole time. Moms need access to safe cannabis. Moms need education on methods of consumption. We need to talk about harm reduction. Families need support in order to talk to their doctors about their cannabis use. We need safe spaces, as melanated women, without threat of our babies being taken from us for cannabis consumption.

Black women deserve the same respect as other women who use cannabis while pregnant. In one article I read recently, it described white women reportedly "using marijuana cigarettes" and Black women as "smoking joints" during pregnancy. That language there is fucked up. Black women are criminalized for "illicit drug use" during pregnancy and white women are revolutionary hippie moms using the latest alternative medicine, or trailblazing into a male-dominated industry. Not while I'm here. I'm taking up space. I will be seen and heard on this topic, with the hopes of providing education to break stigmas and stereotypes. We deserve birth equity and cannabis equity at the same damn time.

The prohibition of cannabis and the war on drugs directly impacted Black women and our families. I believe that cannabis can potentially restore our health and well-being individually and collectively. Becoming a doula, for me, is about selflessly caring for birthing people, being nonjudgmental of people's birth choices, and providing them with or connecting them to evidence based information and education. I'm providing the care that I desperately needed as a first time mom. Unbiased, holistic birth support. I'm creating herb and cannabis infused goods for the body, bath, and home especially catering to women's health, pregnancy, and postpartum. I'll be collaborating with other women run brands in the cannabis space and other birthworkers with the hopes of creating honest dialogue and thorough educational and eventful workshops.

Greetings Joy,

I resubmitted my 5th application (last Saturday) and was able to see a doctor for certification for my condition.

Is there any way to forward my application on so that I'm able to start treatment?

My original application was submitted in June 2018.

Thank you,

Melanie Julion

Cannabis & Pregnancy:
Three Things You Need to Know

I receive a lot of questions about women using cannabis for pregnancy and postpartum related symptoms and for menstrual cramps, body aches, etc. from mamas, doulas, and midwives. There is a lot of misinformation on the internet, so it is no wonder so many women are shy about their consumption. Most of the cannabis industry is marketing its products to young, single males when it's actually mothers who make and influence the health decisions for everyone in her family. I am confident, however, that more research is being done on the benefits of cannabis on women's health and thus more education will follow.

Nevertheless, here are **THREE** important things you need to know (there's more!):

1. There is not sufficient research to prove the benefits or harm of cannabis on pregnant women and/or on her unborn baby! However, there is medical evidence that has proven that even when the fetus is as tiny as two cells, it has an Endocannabinoid System with receptors that binds to cannabinoids present in cannabis, such as CBD, to promote the growth and function of other body systems. Many pregnant women who have used cannabis during pregnancy have gone on to birth healthy, full term babies. In places like Jamaica, for example, women have reported heavy use of cannabis during pregnancy with no complications or side effects. The other research that does exist, is highly flawed.

2. If you are considering using cannabis while you are pregnant, talk to your doctor or midwife. If you do use cannabis and you are pregnant, practice safe consumption. If you choose not to, that's great. Don't shame other women for their choice, opinion or thoughts about using cannabis while pregnant, especially if you lack proper information.

3. Many women have experienced relief from common pregnancy concerns such as pain relief, nausea, insomnia, hormonal and mood

imbalances, the list goes on. People who are pregnant and are unable to take prescription medication to manage their mental health, also use cannabis to treat depression and anxiety. It's often the healthier alternative. Keep in mind also, that using cannabis requires making an informed decision, like many other decisions that women have to make during pregnancy and it is important to talk to your doctor. If your doctor is not aware of your consumption and for whatever reason does a drug test on you and your baby, the situation may not end well. However, if you are informed, and practicing safe consumption: a registered patient, using organic cannabis, medicating with an appropriate strain and application then there would be no reason for a doctor to suspect child negligence or drug abuse.

If you need assistance talking to your doctors about safe cannabis use during pregnancy and postpartum, I offer this service to my birth doula clients and to people interested in becoming registered medical cannabis patients. It can be a pretty intense conversation, especially when your provider isn't supportive (or informed) and it's good to be prepared with factual information about cannabis void of the stereotypes and misinformation often directed at Black mothers.

To learn what cannabis strains, products, and methods of consumption that work best for you and your lifestyle, schedule a consultation with The Cannabis Doula, Certified Cannabis Consultant, HypnoDoula & Childbirth Educator.

Becoming A Medical Cannabis Patient

Exactly a month ago, I sat in the doctor's office with my fiancé and our two sons, as a woman I'd just met tells me that a biopsy and ultrasound of my thyroid and neck was suspicious of thyroid cancer. I smiled. Surely, she'd made a mistake.

A week prior, I had brought in a CT of my neck from three years ago when I had first noticed the lumps there. I thought it was due to swelling from having several wisdom teeth extracted and thought nothing more of it. Until now. The lumps are still here. Not painful, but somewhat noticeable. Still, I thought maybe it had something to do with giving birth or breastfeeding. After all, our body's change so much & postpartum thyroiditis is a thing. So I went to Johns Hopkins, I scheduled an appointment with otolaryngology. The surgeon did a scope of my throat and didn't notice anything unusual. After viewing my CT scans he tell us that we should probably prepare ourselves for The C-word. "I see it all the time, I'm not worried. If it is cancer, don't worry, we can have a small surgery to remove the thyroid. It's the common procedure in this case," He says and gave me the information for an endocrinologist, who apparently only took clients seven months out. With his referral, he assured me, I'd get an appointment the next week.

So here we are, sitting in a small examine room, as this woman, the endocrinologist, tells me, in otherwise perfect health, the one thing that I never imagined would change my life forever. She goes on and on about the surgery, the 4-week recovery, and the radioactive iodide that would follow. Plus, the hormone pills and lifelong doctor visits after that. The entire time, I'm smiling, half listening trying to keep Mars and Messiah entertained. Completely unbothered by the news. In fact, I thought and still think, the whole thing was hilarious. Serious, but funny, and sad in the way providers attempt to plant fear in patients in order to get their consent to thousand dollar surgeries and treatment plans— even though natural healing and cures exist. So, I just smiled.

Before now, I've used cannabis to treat self-diagnosed anxiety, depression, and maybe PTSD. Nausea and insomnia, and whatever else. But I never really considered myself as a cannabis patient. I gained cannabis knowledge and experience in the industry with the humble intentions of inspiring others to use cannabis to heal themselves! My use of cannabis has been mostly recreational with medicinal benefits. Now, everything is different.

When I told the doctor of my intention to use medical cannabis, his response was the generic response that most doctors are required by hospital protocol to give, as to be expected. I will be using cannabis to treat thyroid cancer. I'm currently in the process of becoming a medical cannabis patient in my state. While I know there is a lot of fear, and shame, and whatever else associated with cancer, and with cannabis use, that often leads people into fear based thinking—I am excited for the opportunity to use RSO, a highly concentrated cannabis oil, along with other herbs (plus an alkaline vegan diet, fasting, and exercise) to heal my thyroid and my body, mind, & spirit. & most importantly, to share my journey—because clearly my throat chakra is all fucked up!

Surgery, especially removing such an important organ as the thyroid, is not an option for me and will never be the best choice, regardless of what Western medicine diagnoses. While I know many people are unaware of the healing power of herbs and of cannabis, especially in killing cancerous cells and improving thyroid function, I'm conscious! Healing is a natural, mind-body-spirit phenomenon so I'll be healing and balancing naturally. "How can you heal if you've never healed?" the universe asked me, in the midst of my shame and embarrassment. So, I'm healing. & Happy.

I'm grateful. I was challenged originally with whether or not to tell people. I was crippled slightly due to the fear of shame and embarrassment. People tend to plant their worse fear onto others and often neglect evidence based information in the process. There are so many people who, would never question their doctor, their doctor's diagnosis or treatment and even asking for a second opinion is blasphemy. For them, there is nothing to research, no alternative to consider because "whatever the doctor says, goes." I'm not one of those people. I don't ever want to put on a facade like everything is perfect and these moments aren't challenging but my happiness is absolute, not relative. I've had far worse moments, and have overcome triumphantly a whole lot of shit that many people should never live through. I'm not interested in being an advocate for surviving cancer or fighting cancer in any traditional sense. Surviving, fighting, and treating cancer is not healing or curing it! I also don't want to be quiet about the fact that more people (young, Black, and women) are being diagnosed with cancer and dying from carcinogens in our environment and in our foods while cures like cannabis, are being suppressed and stigmatized, especially in Black communities.

Becoming a medical cannabis patient will make me a better caregiver! I'll be crafting my own medicine, herbal infusions, and edibles to heal MY body. I hope to be transparent throughout this entire time, to aid in my healing. I'll be sharing my journey here, and doing videos and demonstrations. I'll be hosting educational workshops and events to elevate cannabis healing and break the stigma associated with cannabis. Join me!

How are you using cannabis to heal?

Cannabis to Address
Maternal Mortality

Is cannabis the answer to the rising Black maternal mortality crisis?

After my beautiful surprise of a home birth with my first son, Messiah, I was rushed to the nearest hospital where I had to get stitches for third degree lacerations (including what I know now as the Husband Stitch) and where I spent the first two days postpartum. It was ridiculous. We barely ate or slept the entire time. My first shower and trip to the bathroom was a horrible experience in a sterile, cold environment with nurses coming in and out every two hours. What I remember most from that experience is when I asked the nurses/doctors for pain medication, and they told me the only two options I had were, Tylenol or Oxycodon. I was in a lot of pain and I knew that Tylenol would be of little help. I was in so much pain, not from giving birth, but from these stitches that the OB violently sutured. I knew from childbirth education classes, that narcotics interfere with breastfeeding and bonding, and isn't safe for the baby. So I couldn't understand then why a highly addictive narcotic was being offered to women immediately after giving birth.

Our body's works really hard after birth regulating hormones, contracting the uterus, producing breastmilk, releasing the placenta, allowing us to love on and care for our babies. If women are given addictive drugs at such a sensitive time, the risk of dependency is so much greater! I'm thankful that I knew better, that I knew to look up the names of the drugs they offered me, and that I was able to deny them even though I was in so much pain and even after being repeatedly offered the narcotics. Still, however, I suffered in pain and in silence after giving birth for a long time because I refused harmful pharmaceuticals.

This shocking reality is why I advocate for cannabis consumption during postpartum, especially. Cannabis works by binding to receptors in our body and alleviates the cause of pain, it doesn't numb the pain like synthetic chemicals. Plus, there are no side effects. Safe cannabis consumption is important for pregnant & nursing mothers and we deserve access and education for natural pain relief to aid any discomfort related to pregnancy and childbirth.

Traditionally, cannabis in various methods of consumption, was used to induce labor, to speed up a stalled birth, for a faster and easier birth, and to stop hemorrhage, as well as treating symptoms related to postpartum depression and psychosis.

So to answer the question, can cannabis be used to address maternal mortality?

For me and more many other families who choose cannabis, the answer is yes.

The Black History of Cannabis

Everything has a Black history. Like most other things, Cannabis history has been largely distorted based on who writes the books and the laws. Cannabis has been a part of Black culture since the time of our ancient ancestors, and the racially motivated prohibition of cannabis and the War on Drugs continues to stifle the growth of Black families and communities for generations.

Here is a brief (messy) history of cannabis:

Cannabis use can be traced back to Ancient Africa and Ancient Egyptian societies, then spread throughout Mesopotamia, Persia, Asia and India. Hemp was used for all kinds of things, especially medicinal and spiritual practices. The psychoactive effects of smoking cannabis were well known by our ancestors. Cannabis was traded across continents as hemp seeds traveled with enslaved Africans, and indentured Indians, all over the world. Africans often braided seeds in their hair during capture, enslavement, and human trafficking as a means to keep their land, food, and traditions sacred. This is how hemp came to the Americas and the Caribbeans. Cannabis grows naturally in Western Africa and parts of Asia. Hemp was then cultivated all over the U.S., especially in southern states like Kentucky that relied heavily on slave labor. Hemp was a cash crop and was imported, exported, and traded all over the world. Except in places like Africa, among Black populations, hemp plantations and cannabis plants were destroyed and its use was associated with witchcraft and evil.

"In Germany, France, England, the United States, and Switzerland, numerous drugs whose main ingredient was hemp were prescribed by trained physicians from about 1845 to about 1951. Among the indications listed were: weak labor contractions, rheumatism, sleep disorders, chronic uterine bleeding not associated with menstruation, colic, cramps, cholera, asthma, lung depression, gastric neurosis, dyspepsia, migraine headache, coughs, bronchitis, excessive milk secretions, carcinoma, difficult labor, vomiting during pregnancy, urethra deficiencies, women's disorders, gonorrhea, neurasthenia, debility, headache, tuberculosis, lung diseases, dysmenorrhea, gout, uratic diathesis, gall-heart-burn, stomachache, enteritis, flatulence, nausea, lack of appetite, constipation, kidney and bladder disorders, inflammations, cystitis, eczema, whooping cough, anemia, overexertion, anxiety states, tiredness, night sweats, hardening of the arteries, dizziness, nervousness, rachitis; in short: Scientific medicine utilized cannabis as a universal remedy!" [via Hemp museum]

Cultivating cannabis (hemp) is such a labor intensive process, that enslaved labor was the only way hemp plantations could produce enough to profit as there were very little agricultural machines in the industry at the time. Slaveowners (often called farmers or planters) were mandated to grow hemp in many states. Let's be clear, the slaves were growing and tending to the cannabis in the fields. Not the white land owners, or slaveowners, such as Thomas Jefferson, or George Washington. Slaveowners apparently used cannabis to pacify their slaves and often allowed enslaved Africans (referred to as Laborers now in some texts) to grow their own cannabis, often referring to it as the nigger crop. In fact enslaved men who were especially skilled in the cultivation of hemp, were so highly sought after, they were of most expensive enslaved persons for sale during this time.

On the reverse, stereotypes associated with smoking cannabis spread as white people saw it as a drug that made enslaved Africans "think that they are on the same level as white men" and a drug that "made white women sexually attracted to Black men." With slave labor being outlawed, many plantations continued to produce hemp with labor from Black sharecroppers long after slavery was outlawed and enslaved people were told of their freedom.

Mexican immigrants who brought smokable hemp, aka marijuana with them into southern states around the time of the Mexican Revolution in 1910s-20s, caused more white fear and even more of a reason to outlaw cannabis use. Marijuana is a term Mexicans used to disguise their sacred use of the cannabis plant within the context of the Christian religion, that was later used as a racist term by white people. Racial propaganda surrounding marijuana began to spread, mostly by Harry Anslinger, who at the time was the head of what is now the DEA, who specifically sought to invoke fear in white women. White discomfort and fear of smoking marijuana became mainstream, through movies, cartoons, and

241

media publications depicting Black men as criminals and devils smoking. Not long after the Marijuana Tax Act in 1942, that required hemp cultivators to have special permits, farmers began to import hemp, and more cheaper alternatives, ultimately ending the cultivation of hemp in the U.S.

While cannabis culture remained underground in Black and Brown communities alike, Black artists like Billie Holiday and many others, were publicly targeted by Anslinger for their cannabis consumption. In the 1930s, Black jazz musicians, writers, and activists during the Harlem Renaissance used marijuana for artistic expression and freedom from racial turmoil. Music about the benefits of cannabis can be noted across all genres of Black music. From the 1930s blues and jazz movement, to reggae in the 1950s and 60s, then to hip hop from the 1970s and 80s to present day. In fact, reggae music and our struggle for equality and peace is what inspired white Hippie culture of the 1960s & 70s to bring cannabis into white mainstream American culture which then brought potential legalization of cannabis to the forefront, and the emergence of a cannabis industry in California, and other states.

Cannabis was used widely among Black peace advocates, civil rights activists, and Black revolutionaries and was another reason for Ronald Reagan to see cannabis as a national threat. Meanwhile, as police and government officials continued to enforce this War on Drugs, first declared by President Nixon, they strictly targeted cannabis related crimes specifically, and in Black and Brown communities disproportionately. Hundreds of thousands of Black and Brown people, men, women, and children are jailed for cannabis distribution or possession, and low level non-violent drug offenses every year—stripped of their rights to vote and the right to a just livelihood because of racially motivated cannabis prohibition. Generations upon generations of Black families and communities have been stifled as jails have filled at alarming rates. The War on Drugs allowed for the consumption of the most harmful drugs, like crack and heroin, in Black communities (and meth and cocaine in white communities) as misleading cannabis propaganda spread. Black families may never recover from the damage caused by cannabis prohibition and propaganda.

After cannabis prohibition spread around the world, however, the U.S. government soon began to fund its own federal medical cannabis research in Israel, supplied its own medical cannabis patients, and to this day continues to research cannabis for medical purposes while claiming it has no medical benefits thus continuing to classify cannabis as a Schedule 1 Drug. It was through this research of THC in the 1990s, the main psychoactive cannabinoid found in marijuana, that our endogenous cannabinoid Anandamide and our entire Endocannabinoid System was discovered! Our Endocannabinoid System is responsible for maintaining homeostasis in our bodies, and regulating other vital processes such as mood, memory, pain, and more.

With more states legalizing cannabis, wealthy white men are getting rich from dispensaries and other cannabis businesses in the now legal blossoming cannabis industry. Especially those with money to afford licenses, land, and labor. A new market and industry is being marketed to rich, white families, and their dogs, of course. While Black families, brown, and low income families are still being torn apart and criminalized; damaged from generations of abuse due to the prohibition of cannabis.

This brief messy history of cannabis in America is why Black people should take OWNERSHIP in this industry. As of right now, people who apply for a dispensary license must have hundreds of dollars in liquid assets, legal and financial counsel. As a means to diversify the industry, special points are given to largely white male owners for hiring minority employees and managers as a means to give Black people equity and diversity. This is not just or equitable. Black communities are owed reparations in the cannabis industry. Black people are owed reparations for the damage caused by prohibition and a racist drug war. As I mentioned previously, cannabis cultivation is labor intensive. Black and Brown people are only being sought after for specific roles in the industry: employees. Black cannabis business owners and entrepreneurs are not being funded, and are expected to meet impossible requirements! Black people should have ownership in this industry, because like most industries in this country, it was built off the backs of enslaved labor, at the expense of our culture, families and community.

So when you hear that cannabis has a complicated, complex, messy, difficult history in the Unites States, or anything to that regard, I hope this helps you to understand why simply discussing social equity in the cannabis industry is not enough; we are due reparations.

Tips for supporting Black/Brown cannabis equity, and cannabis reparations for a Black communities:

- Buy weed from Black women.
- Support local social equity programs.
- Donate/Invest in Black-owned cannabis brands and businesses.
- Be vocal.
- Support cannabis education and caregiver services for survivors of the war on drugs, including elders and chronically ill people.
- Advocate for the expungement of all nonviolent cannabis-related offenses and criminal records of Black and Brown people in your state.
- Ensure that families are not separated due to cannabis use.
- Return stolen land to Black and Indigenous communities.
- Remove financial barriers required to obtain cannabis licenses.
- Release all political prisoners and enslaved people from for-profit prisons.
- Pay reparations to the descendants of enslaved African people who cultivated cannabis as a cash crop, and the descendants of African people and communities who were directly targeted, killed, and imprisoned due to racism and the war on drugs.

Hi Joy,

I resubmitted my patient application a month ago and have not heard back. Can you please provide me with feedback as I need to start my cannabis treatment for thyroid cancer. I am willing to come in person to verify any information.

Thank you

Melanie

My Dream for Melanated Mothers

Mothering is such a transformational experience and to be honest, most of our mothering starts long before we birth babies of our own. So I'm thankful for that. For everything and everyone that has taught me how to mother. I'm the coolest mom, due to some really cool moms I know. Happy Mother's Day!

- Black people's children have the same opportunities to grow up as white people's children. (i.e. not be unjustly killed by police/vigilantes for being Black)
- Black women mother instinctually and spiritually, free of fear and generational trauma
- We make choices for the care of our own children without commentary or critical gaze from non-Black people or perceived authority figures
- We breastfeed, if we choose or have healthy alternatives
- We love who we choose, and how we choose
- We have access to safe, affordable, clean housing for our children
- We have clean water for ourselves, our families, and our children
- We have quality, affordable childcare for our children
- We have quality educational institutions or access to quality teaching material to educate our children
- We birth in peace and free of trauma
- We birth without fear of our children being taken away or dying
- We have access to fresh fruit and vegetables for our families
- We have access to safe playgrounds, community centers, pools, organized play and recreation
- We gather, in sisterhood and community with each other, to raise our children as a village, with genuine love and respect for Black life and family
- We live free of white supremacy, white insecurity, and white fragility.
- We have access to traditional healing medicine and remedies, medical cannabis, herbs, and other natural holistic remedies for the sustained health and well-being of our bodies and families

A short list I felt compelled to put together for my hopes, dreams, affirmations for Black mothers & babies. Goals for me to keep in mind as I do this work and live this life.

What is your dream for melanated mothers?

Three Steps to Shatter the Stigma
by The Cannabis Doula

1. Learn the physical, and spiritual benefits of cannabis for women, the best consumption method for you and how to incorporate cannabis into your individual and unique daily wellness plan

2. Grow to embrace the healing potential of cannabis, connect with other women and mothers who consume in a safe and supportive community.

3. Evolve. Become a member of the cannabis mom collective and join The Cannabis Doula for our Meditate, Meet & Greet, a cannabis infused meditation session for mothers, our Revolutionary Motherhood Birth Circles, and cannabis healing seshs.

Cannabis: A Healthy Alternative to Commonly Used Medications in Maternity Suites

I want to take you back to a moment that you may have heard me mention. A moment that was traumatic for me. When I was offered and refused narcotics (opioids) for the severe pain that I experienced from having stitches for third degree lacerations after what was a beautiful and unplanned precipitous homebirth with my first son. I was in labor and gave birth in less than an hour, which is not uncommon for moms who use cannabis throughout pregnancy. Quick & easy, pain-free birth. However, I spent my first two days as a new mother in a maternity suite at the nearest hospital barely able to move, walk, or use the bathroom without pain.

My pain was not from giving birth. In fact, my birth was exhilarating. I was in pain largely due to a mean ass OB who violently sutured me up and was even more violent and dismissive toward me for refusing opioids, Pitocin, and IVs (plus vaccinations and all other newborn interventions). Truth is, I planned for a natural water birth at the birth center where I was receiving prenatal care, but when I called them to tell the midwife that I was in labor, she told me to call her back because I was a first-time mom and we usually have long labors. So, I had my baby 30 minutes later on daddy's couch and ended up in the hospital's maternity suite for aftercare.

Anyway, I'm particularly critical of hospitals, for reasons unbeknownst to me but I can say is probably due to generational trauma which is why I had no plan to give birth there. I've often come to find that the people who work in hospitals are only following orders and protocols that are largely outdated, not evidence-based, and in complete opposition to what's best for mama and baby, and often times rooted in racism and classism. How unfortunate for most doctors and nurses who really think they are helping people.

(Disclaimer: I love good doctors and nurses who advocate for their patients, and who go above and beyond hospital protocols, like the good doctors at Grey-Sloan Memorial Hospital, whose doctors are well-known recipients of the Harper Avery/Catherine

Fox award for excellence in medicine...a little Grey's Anatomy humor to lighten this up a bit?)

So yesterday, I was going through some old paperwork and found my discharge papers from this hospital experience. I often like to look over my discharge papers to see if I've missed anything that I didn't know or see prior. In this packet, I find listed all the medications that the nurses gave me and the medications that they use commonly in maternity suites. And what do you know, oxycodone was listed as being given to me twice, two different dosages. Strange, I thought. I know I declined, repeatedly. I made it clear that I was breastfeeding (and that I was a doula and I knew the effects of narcotics on nursing babies and mamas) so why is this listed? Did they give me oxycodone without my permission? I don't fucking know. But I do know that moms who are on Medicaid are prescribed opioids more often and I was receiving Medicaid at the time. Did they list it just to get money from Medicaid on my behalf? I don't fucking know. But I do know that something ain't right. So I did more digging.

Opioids are commonly prescribed to pregnant and breastfeeding women in spite of the known negative risks, including opioid withdrawals in newborn babies, issues breastfeeding, and the list goes on. According to the FDA, severe and persistent pain that is not effectively treated during pregnancy can result in depression, anxiety, and high blood pressure in the mother. But are opioids the solution to the pain that women experience in pregnancy and postpartum? Hell fucking no, is the answer to that. We have to be really honest, our country is facing an opioid problem. This we know, but we've never stopped to think about how this crisis is impacting pregnant women and babies; the most vulnerable in our communities. And the reason we haven't done so, is because these drugs are making hospitals lots of money. There is a reason doctors are prescribing opioids. There is a high chance that once a patient fills their opioid prescription, they will continue to refill their prescription. Opioids are highly addictive. Do they work to eliminate the source of the pain? Or do they just numb the symptoms related to the pain temporarily? Big questions, that we already know the answers to.

Black mothers are dying. We need safe alternatives. Like yesterday.

sounds trumpet

Thankfully, Queen Cannabis has our back.

Cannabis, in its various forms of consumption, is a safer alternative to common pharmaceutical medications found on maternity suites. Yup. I told you cannabis was used traditionally for women, right? From pain, to blood pressure, hemorrhoids, itching, cracked nipples, infection, digestion, constipation, and the list goes on. I'm supporting families who are no longer interested in being misinformed by care providers who have invested interest in pharmaceutical companies. For families who are interested in natural alternatives that have no negative side effects on their babies or their breastmilk. For moms who choose cannabis, the possibility of healing all of the changes that come with motherhood—physically, spiritually, mentally, and emotionally, cannabis is truly promising.

For more information or to learn about cannabis alternatives to common medications used during pregnancy and postpartum, contact The Cannabis Doula to schedule a consultation. I provide clients with education and research to help inform your doctors and family about the benefits of cannabis, I provide support and tips to avoid negative interactions with Child Protective Services, and importantly, I provide cannabis caregiver services to help families learn to prepare cannabis medication including topicals, tinctures, infused oils, edibles, capsules, and more that can be used to aid moms from pregnancy to postpartum and beyond.

Dear Melanie,

Your application to register as a Patient with MMCC has been approved.

May 31, 2019

Thank you for following me on this journey. If you've been following me for some time, you've watched me grow, birth two babies, and so much more. If I make it look easy, it's not! But it is truly rewarding. At 29, this is the life I worked so hard to manifest over the last five years. I went from working a toxic corporate job, to growing cannabis, then becoming a mom, a doula, and childbirth educator and really living in my purpose which is so heavily tied to cannabis and turning the poison of our lives into medicine to heal ourselves and our families.

It's an honor and a privilege to me to hold space for women and families. Especially for women who choose cannabis as a healthier alternative to pharmaceuticals and other medical interventions.

I love cannabis for recreational purposes but I'm also a medical cannabis patient. Cannabis doesn't make me a better mom, it allows me to show up as my full authentic self, which is naturally a dope ass mom.

I use cannabis for depression, anxiety, and PTSD related to childhood trauma and workplace trauma. I used cannabis during two pregnancies, childbirth, & postpartum and while breastfeeding both my babies—to treat nausea, pain, insomnia, mood imbalances, and everything else. I will also be using cannabis oil/RSO (along with other herbs, a mostly alkaline vegan diet, and exercise—thank you Dr. Sebi) to heal thyroid cancer.

We have a lot to talk about.
Let's #ShatterTheStigma together.

Use Your B.R.A.I.N.
to Make Informed Decisions

This strategy can be used for any medical decision, especially during pregnancy & childbirth.

Medical interventions and surgeries, no matter how common they may be, do not come without risks. Narcotics (opioids like codeine, oxycodone, Percocet, etc), even acetaminophen and Tylenol should not be taken without determining the risks. Why are doctors prescribing opioids to pregnant women when it's widely known that these drugs are dangerous, addictive, and should not be used during pregnancy or while breastfeeding? Babies are being born addicted to narcotics, they suffer from symptoms of withdrawal for the first months of life, have issues nursing, sleeping, etc. and then are expected to get vaccines! Yikes. .

It is especially important for birthing people to have safe access to safer alternatives to opioids in the management of pain and other symptoms related to pregnancy, childbirth, and postpartum. This is why I advocate for safe cannabis consumption for moms. Cannabis is a safer alternative, and has no dangerous side effects to mom or baby.

A few months ago, I used this same strategy to decide whether I'd have surgery to have my thyroid removed upon being diagnosed with thyroid cancer. If I'd decided to have the surgery instead of researching alternatives, possible risks, and long term consequences of removing my thyroid I would be, without a doubt, fighting for my life at this very moment. If I'd listen to the fears of others, especially family, I wouldn't be able to live or function without having to use pharmaceutical drugs every day. That's not the life I want to live nor anyone should have to live when our bodies are perfectly capable of healing themselves (and birthing babies) without much intervention.

If you are pregnant and or breastfeeding and considering using cannabis, use this strategy to make the best informed decision for you and your baby!

June 8, 2019

The Women Grow Leadership Summit was amazing, of course.

I'm still blown away. I met so many amazing women, so many amazing Black women who have dedicated their lives to cannabis wellness and education. Hella inspiring! I connected with local cultivators, entrepreneurs, registered nurses, sex educators, a pediatrician, and an OB-GYN, who decided to quit their respective practices and focus on cannabis education, advocacy, and care especially within our community.

Women are powerful.
We need each other.
We have the solutions.

This weekend allowed us to connect the dots on ideas and plans to really forward conversations on shattering the stigma related to cannabis in all aspects. I'm so thankful for the women who shared their experiences and intimate parts of their lives, especially the women who shared the panel with me on the conversation of Cannabis & Family Wellness.

I'm so excited for the work to come.

June 19, 2019

Let's Shatter The Stigma.

Let's talk about weed! Cannabis can be used to heal our bodies, our families, and our communities. Do you smoke or use cannabis in any other form? Would/Do you use cannabis for medical purposes?

I've been using cannabis for nine years. I started working in the cannabis industry, growing medical cannabis for patients in 2015. It took me almost nine months to become a medical cannabis patient in my state. I'm using cannabis for depression, anxiety, PTSD, & thyroid cancer. It is a privilege to be able to go to the store to buy weed, and most people that I know live in places where they don't have access to legal, quality marijuana, especially people who could most benefit from it–are still stigmatized and criminalized for using it.

Since today is Juneteenth, it's a good time to talk about how enslaved Africans grew hemp/cannabis on plantations in this country largely contributing to the growth of hemp as a cash crop! For centuries, before the government ultimately outlawed its use, largely for racist and prejudice beliefs about cannabis, Africans used cannabis for healing and spiritual reasons, and for food and fiber. Hemp seeds were spread all over the world as they traveled with enslaved Africans in the slave trade who hoped to keep a part of their homeland and themselves by hiding the seeds in their hair and clothing. I'm happy that enslaved Africans were able to keep their use of cannabis and hemp as tradition, so we honor our ancestors every time we flame up. Asé.

Happy Juneteenth.

Today is also a good day to talk about reparations in the form of equity and ownership (not just employment) in the cannabis industry.

June 21, 2019

A recent post by the American College of Obstetricians and Gynecologists is exactly why cannabis education for birthing families is so important. It's important for pregnant people to have access to adequate, and accurate cannabis education and research, and as more pregnant women are reporting using cannabis it also becomes extremely important that families have access to adequate support and care in their cannabis consumption. I encourage all moms, and anyone interested in cannabis use during pregnancy to read this article and play close attention to the language. The disclaimers before and after the article, the highlighted amendments, and the references. There is enough research on cannabis use during pregnancy for women and families to make informed decisions. There is also misinformation, propaganda, flawed and biased research based on racist stereotypes out there as well. I'm working with local dispensaries, hospitals, and birthing centers to dispel the misinformation and fear on cannabis use during pregnancy!

During my Healthy Cannabis Consumption Workshop, I'll be teaching families and birth workers about how to dissect the research on cannabis use during pregnancy and how to use evidence based research and cannabis science to make an informed choice. This infographic is misleading, based on flawed research, and the opinions of their council, not the most recent evidence, as their website directly states. I'm so disappointed that they would post this, as so many women are turning to cannabis as a safer alternative, and after the World Health Organization recently stated that CBD is a safe to use during pregnancy. I would love to hear your thoughts on this. *Is a recommendation from ACOG important in your decision to use cannabis during pregnancy, or suggest it to others?*

This weekend, I'll be joining with local cannabis moms, doulas, and birthworkers for an intimate conversation to shatter the stigma on this and cultivate a village to provide support to cannabis consuming families.

June 27, 2019

I love being a mom.

I especially love visiting libraries and parks in the middle of the day and going for walks and other adventures. I love my boys and I'm so thankful that I get to mother the way I choose, in a world that constantly tells us what to do and how to live. I can't believe I have a one year old and two and a half year old!

I can't even imagine transitioning into motherhood without the use of cannabis. It's helped tremendously in managing my emotions, balancing my hormones, and improving my mood. I'm working on building a strong Endocannabinoid System and using cannabis is just one part of that.

My favorite method of consumption lately has been rolling CBD flower, with other herbs. It brings such harmony to my crazy life and allows me to be completely at peace and present in the moment.

Subscribe to The Cannabis Doula on YouTube, I'm sharing all about my recent dispensary visits, taking the boys to the dispensary, and my journey using cannabis to heal and empower women.

July 12, 2019

I often have the urge to reintroduce myself—especially to people who think they know me. Luckily though, most of these people—friends and family—are not a part of my everyday life. I realize now that moving away from them was my way of trying to relieve myself of the responsibility that we each have when we face the people who made us into the person that we've healed or had to do work not to be.

As a person, healing, mentally, physically, and spiritually from past childhood trauma from witnessing domestic violence, from racist/sexist workplace trauma, self-inflicted trauma by succumbing to white supremacist physical attacks with emotion, from being raised with a curse of poverty and a slave mentality, from Post-Traumatic Slave Syndrome, from sexual and emotional violence inflicted on me from men, from the sexual and emotional violence I may have inflicted onto others in my state of weakness and immaturity. I'm healing from the first 29 years of my life. I'm healing my throat chakra from being someone who I was not, for so long. I realize now that in so many relationships, affiliations, and friendships, I could have avoided so much heartache—I could have avoided a society of ill-willed people, vultures, and conformists.

Some lessons have to be learned through living, that's why there aren't any books (or very few) on things that I want to know about.

Truth is, the experience is worth it.

To be able to be where I am now, with a family, two beautiful boys, a growing village, doing what I love educating on babies, books, and cannabis, living in love everyday in connection with the entire universe and guided by my ancestors, elders, and spirit guides. I'm walking the path to enlightenment and to a continual flow of abundance and wealth in the form of monies, land, property, and cannabis.

Honoring Cannabis as A Sacred Herb

I honor the sacred plant cannabis, ganja, weed, marijuana, and all the names she has to take in order to heal others in her natural state—like Black women must do.

I honor the cannabis seeds that traveled from Africa to the Americas, on the bodies, the hair, and clothing of Africans held captive as slaves.

I honor the cannabis grown by enslaved Africans in southern slave plantations in the United States, as a cash crop during slavery.

I honor my ancestors and all Black people who have died, been abused, unjustly tried or imprisoned because of the racist agenda, propaganda, and misinformation surrounding the use and cultivation of cannabis.

To those who currently face racial stigma because of cannabis, those who currently face legal issues or imprisonment because of cannabis May your sacrifice produce great fruit.

I honor cannabis as sacred medicine gifted to us by our ancestors who suffered great atrocities in the cultivation of their sacred herb.

I am grateful.

Setting Intentions With Cannabis

Through the use of cannabis my intention is to:

_____

_____

Through the use of cannabis my intention is to heal: _____

_____

_____

My intention is to grow: _____

My intention is learn:_____

My intention is to evolve through cannabis by_____

_____

_____

Be intentional with your cannabis consumption.
Inhale: Joy, Happiness, and Peace
Exhale: Fear, Anger, and Tension

The cannabis that I consume heals _____

The cannabis that I consume supports me by_____

_____

Tips for best results:
- Incorporate three methods of consumption or more.
- Consistency is key.
- Consume internal and external cannabis applications.
- Consume good, clean, quality cannabis.

July 14, 2019

What hurts the most?

Some would say the emotional pain. But right now—for me it's the bruise that I have on my hips and back, and my head from hitting the floor. I can still feel his hands around my neck, my feet dangled probably one foot from the floor. His hand/ arm fully extended as he choked the shit out of me. For the second time.
Also, the second time he threw me on the ground—at least this time I'm not pregnant.

The impact of my fall yesterday was enough to make me feel like going to urgent care. But mommy duties last night consisted of caring for Mars, after he threw up his entire dinner—right on my yoga mat and in front of my alter. If that wasn't a clear sign from the ancestors—I don't know what is. We have to leave. The crazy part is I don't even remember calling my mom. I would have never imagined, in a million years, that I'd have the courage to be honest about my crumbling relationship. A relationship doomed from the start.

And Patra asked some important questions. She made sure I didn't go to sleep with even the slightest idea that it was my fault. One day she'll know the full story. We come from strong women. I'm thankful for the clarity to be finally moving on.
I welcome love, into my life.
Pure love.

No matter what you do or say no man should ever try to justify hitting a woman.

Does throwing away a bottle of syrup warrant being choked up against a wall? Or being thrown across the room by my head?

In front of my children?

*If he could do all of this while on Facetime with his mom—what is he capable of doing when no one is there?

My stomach still hurts from the impact. I hope I'm not pregnant.
I'm breaking the cycle of domestic violence. Or I'm going to die—there
is no question about it. If I stay, or go back to Jackson, I will die (and
maybe that is what he wants.)

It's weird though.

Because he said he loved me. He was never really here this whole time.

I looked at his IG and thought, wow—I'm just one picture in his life.
I'm a single mention. I birthed two of his children. Every woman before me decided to abort, or miscarried. I birthed him two healthy Black
boys and he beat my ass for throwing his syrup away.

"It's the principle" he said.

I bet she won't do that shit again—I laid up imagining that what he must
have been thinking after all was said, and done.

And me.

I just keep replaying my head hitting the floor.
Messiah's scream. And Mars' silence. Then his "wow" followed by a
burst of tears as his daddy left the house.

I know this won't be the last time I'll be holding them, crying about
daddy. But this will be the last time they cry because daddy hit mommy.

I'm going to urgent care.

Mommy says "no hitting"
But daddy hit mommy.

Mommy says "no yelling"
But daddy yells at mommy.

Mommy says, "Be Kind, please"
But how?
Daddy's not kind to mommy.

July 16, 2019

This has been the craziest couple of days. Yesterday, I decided to go to the emergency room because my head was still hurting. I asked Jackson if he saw how hard I may have hit my head on the floor when he shoved me. He said I hit my head on the metal bar of the chair we have in the living room.

I immediately think of my grandma's aneurysm, from constant domestic abuse she experienced, and my mom, and I know I had to go to the ER for a CT. No brain bleeding—my diagnosis?

"A closed head injury with concussion, headache, and physical assault."

A fucking concussion, g.
Is that a curse? Most definitely.

Which explains why I don't remember calling my mom and telling her, nor do I remember giving the boys a bath that night and on Sunday when I was doing the live conversation on Cannabis & Black Women's Health I couldn't remember the questions that were asked seconds before—hopefully I played it well and still presented thorough information for folks to consider.
But—fuck all that for right now.
My question is…. *What the FUCK am I going to do??*

"It's only going to get worse," the nurses said, "You have to think about your babies." The men at the desk in the express care center of the E.R. at Holy Cross just laughed and shook their heads when they read the paper detailing how I sustained my injuries. "It never fails," one of them said.

In addition to being recently diagnosed with cancer, one nurse said, "wow, all of this has happened to you, as pretty as you are? There must be a bright light surrounding you."

And she gave me a hug before I left that I so desperately needed.

I pray that my ancestors guide me to healing and beautiful, safe, and peaceful home.

I pray in this moment that all financial prosperity be bestowed upon me and my children.

I pray for light.

I pray for truth, justice, and compassion.

I pray for understanding.

I pray for clarity, vision, and voice.

I pray for strength.

I am not a victim. I am not the things men have said about me or done to me.

I pray for sisters who can help me heal and rebuild.

I pray for peace.

The concussion should be clearing up in a few days—I will have clarity.

I pray to the moon, to yemaya and oshun, to guide me and provide me with a beautiful environment, home, and alter to adorn them.

I pray my ancestors will help me do the work to break the cycle of domestic violence, abuse, and disrespect toward women.

July 20, 2019

I am not a victim.
Domestic Violence.
We are both perpetrators,
but I'm the only one
considered a victim.
Am I the only one hurting?
Do I hurt the most?

"This isn't the first time—won't be the last."
"He's probably cheating
And can't handle the emotions."
"You need to go,
You're a dumb bitch if you stay---"

Black love,
"You have to get counseling."
"You stand by your man."
"He needs you."
"The boys need you,
Together."

It'll happen again and again.
Every time the money low,
The bill is due,
The account overdrawn,
The car ticketed, booted, or towed,
The house dirty,
The dishes not washed,
The food not cooked,
The dick not sucked,
The smile not plastered on my face.

While inside I'm slowly dying.

Why shrink?
Why shrink?

July 23, 2019

I feel like I'm dying.
Like my spirit is dying.
Maybe it's a transition.
My spirit is shifting.
Either way—it hurts.

Is Jackson who I think he is?
Has it been an act this whole time?
Has he been abusive this whole time and I've been so head bumped and
in love perhaps I didn't care? Perhaps I thought it was normal because
I had seen and heard so much dysfunction with my parents

Am I knowingly
perpetuating the cycle of domestic violence?

Am I the victim or the perpetrator?
How did I manifest this into my life?

Will I ever be happy again?
Was I ever really happy?
Am I here only for the boys?
Does he love me?
Why is he so mad?

It's been a week and three days since—
Jackson pushed me causing me to fall hit my head on a metal pole of a
chair causing a mild concussion.
He choked me at least two feet from the floor with his arms fully extended. He threw a book at me. He cursed at me, called me names, belittled
me.

Me—the apparent love of his life—for throwing away his syrup.

And the first thing my parents say:

"Melanie, well why did you throw away his syrup?"
"You don't throw people's stuff away."

No– "Are you okay, do you need to leave for a little while, would you like me to get you a room until you sort things out."
No– "Do you feel safe?"
No, nothing.

I sometimes can't believe the family that I come from and the society that made this family what it is. I hate that in spite of all I've attempted to do to have a healthy family, somehow the evil curse of domestic abuse still lurks up in my life. Ruining the very foundation I've belt my life on. So yes–my fucking life is over and I need time to grieve my death.

I don't know how I can get through this.

I don't want to.

I hate Jackson.
And I hate myself even more for being the type of woman that would put up with bullshit for so long.
I'm so sad.
I'm so, so sad.

He thinks we can get through this.
But I know that's not how domestic violence works.
There is no such thing as getting through only breaking up or the cycle will continue.

He hates me too.
He's just really concerned about being a good guy to other people;
Especially his mom.

Is this what I get for dating him
knowing he was raised by a single-mother?
By the time I had realized the complexities of their mother-son dynam-ic– we were already in too deep.

I can never marry into this family.
I will never be good enough for Jackson.

This shit sucks.

Am I speaking death onto our relationship?
Or has he already done that?

He won't respect me if I stay.
I have no control in our relationship.
Why would he want to be with a weak, quiet woman?

Did I mistake him being an asshole with him being abusive?
How did we get here?
What the fuck.
Did I bump my head a long time ago and I'm just now waking up to bullshit?

Is this the "get out" moment?

"It'll only get worse," they say
or am I the dumb bitch
who decides to stay?

I break generational curses.

Curses of domestic violence and abuse of all kinds.
It is rooted in slavery.
I release it now.

I heal my body, mind, and spirit from the trauma and pain of domestic violence and abuse.
I release it now.

I heal all others from the pain and trauma of intimate partner violence, domestic abuse, violence, and trauma. Emotional abuse, mental and spiritual abuse, financial and economic abuse inflicted on Black women and children. I release it now.

I release from my life any person who is knowingly or unknowingly causing me pain, harm, and danger. I release every person now who does not serve me.

I can no longer move through this life with no money, assets, or property. I release the spirit and curse of poverty. I release it now.

I release the spirit of lack and hunger. I release all brokenness.

I am financially and spiritually rich.

Celebration.

I release my former self.
I truly am the master of my fate.
I am so thankful for I finally know who I am and from whom I come!

I come from root women, healers, and nurturers.

I come from strong women. Brave women. Bold women.

I over-stand why I made the choices I've made and why I love the way
I do. In order to break curses, we have to heal the spirit with the spirit.
The spirit of our foremothers. I am healing my womb and womb of my
mother's mother. And my mother.

I praise my ancestors.

Grams (my great grandma)
Mary Francis Evans Love Robinson- Collins
Self-taught Midwife in Arkansas
Sweet, Stern, Determined, Loving, Kind, and Humble.

July 30, 2019

Ellegua – Oshun – Yemaya,

I resort to your protection and in my faith I offer this light that shall burn every Tuesday.

Comfort me in my difficulties and intercede for me and my family that we will be able to hold the vastness of the universe in our hearts and be provided for in all our necessities. I beseech you to have infinite pity in regard to the favors I ask of you.

1. _____
2. _____
3. _____

I pray that I may be able to overcome all difficulties as you did the dragon at your feet.

Asé
Asé
Asé

I accept wealth!
$ MONEY $
I dance for oshun and yemaya!

All my goals will come to be with the financial abundance that I will receive!

Prospering Business
A House
Land
Sisterhood
So Shall it be!
Breaking Generational Curses!

Money Flows To Me Freely

July 30, 2019

Breaking generational curses and releasing generational trauma like everything involves healing the mind, body, and spirit. In my youth, I thought that I would be able to learn about issues that negatively impacted Black families—issues like domestic violence, poor access of education, health, and adequate housing. I'd learn the causes and how to prevent future children from experiencing things that I'd experienced and seen growing up as a Black girl on the south side of Chicago—I'd learn all of this as a means of preventing these things from manifesting in my own life and the life of my children.

This retrograde has broken me open in so many ways. Everything that manifests in the physical is also present in the mind and the spirit. You can learn all there is to know about the physical cause of an illness but until you address the spirit and the root of the illness, curse, or trauma, you will never heal. Everything that I've experienced recently is only me repeating the same lessons over and over again, but this time was the final lesson. And I finally over-stand. I didn't think I'd make it through this last month, in fact these last few months have been really hard for me. But I'm determined to break generational curses and trauma in my family—trauma caused by domestic violence and abuse against women and children in my family.

I can't even express in words some of the trauma that I experienced as a result of witnessing all forms of domestic violence growing up, but I refuse to continue the cycle by being silent and allowing trauma to dictate my relationships. I'm doing the spiritual work required to break the curse and live abundantly.

I'm thankful, I was reminded of the root women I come from!

Our ancestors have given us so many wonderful gifts so that we can heal and grow. As I'm using cannabis to heal the physical and mental manifestations of the trauma I've experienced, I'm also using cannabis as a sacred herb for healing my spirit and connecting with my ancestors and guides to break generational trauma and release negative energy that has never served me, or the women in my family.

Black Moon | July 31, 2019

Thank you for guiding me through this mercury retrograde.
Divine Spirit, I honor you
and trust
that I am on the path
toward my blessing.
I am on the path
to receiving
my dream home,
and living the life
I've always dreamed
of with my happy,
healthy, loving, family.

I trust the process
and I surrender
my ego and allow you
to move through
and speak through me.

Break open my throat chakra.

I welcome a newness
and a wealth that I've never seen!
And I thank you and
dance in celebration with oshun and yemaya.

August 1st

I am a Cannabis Sommelier.

Very impressive.
Thank you divine for your many blessings.

I am learning tarot with a Voodoo priestess.
Blessings, Blessings, Blessings!

I attract all of my ancestors knowledge!
I am Divine.
I am The All.
I attract all that I am.
I am melanin.
I am peace.

I am the living manifestation of our glorious ancestors
and the hard work–the blood, sweat, and tears,
of the elders.

It's time for me to go.
I think my time on the east coast is over.

August 2nd

I'm reflective.
Really seeing people for who they are now.
I finally understand what
Brother Pete was talking about when he lectured me on *Games People Play.*

Bad vibes.
I can feel them
I can feel ill-intentions coming
my way
from other women;
especially Jackson's mom.
and I guess they've always been there.
It just sucks.
I always thought that the mom and the son's wife were supposed to click instantly. And anything else is a bad sign; a sign to RUN.

If his mom doesn't like me and he loves his mom, there is no limit to the things she'll say and do to make me look like shit to her son.

If he has an unhealthy relationship with his mom, he'll listen to her and start to despise me in order to please her. He'll eventually seek out other women that his mom will like better or who is more like his mom than me.

If he has a healthy relationship with his mom, he'll kindly tell her to shut the fuck up, that his wife is queen, and the only one for him and she'll have to respect that or don't be apart of their village.

It's either the first option or the second and it's usually very clear to see. Men have very complicated relationships with their mothers and it sucks because it's usually the other women that end up hurt when unhealthy mother-son relationships exist.

I pray healing for them and release any man/woman from my life who doesn't respect me, my mission, my spirit. I release anyone, friend or

family that tends to do me harm or speak negatively about me. I release
everyone who has knowingly and unknowingly cursed me or hexed me.
Make dead their spirit.

Let no man or woman
stand in the way of my
blessings of wealth,
fortune, and abundance.

Let them instead
stand in awe
and praise of my *magic.*

"A woman in harmony
with her spirit is like a river flowing.
She goes where she will without pretense
and arrives at her destination
prepared to be herself and only herself."

- Toni Morrison

August 6, 2019

Our beloved Toni Morrison
has joined the ancestors.

Gratitude.

May your work continue through me.
All praises.

Mars' first trip to the theaters was to view your documentary just last month. *We felt you.*

What can I even say other than thank you!

For The Bluest Eye, the book I used to host my first book club.
For Tar Baby.
Thank you for Sula! It changed my life.
Thank you so much for Beloved, the book that shaped my outlook on Black motherhood.
Thank you for Song of Solomon, it taught me how to fly.
Thank you for James Baldwin's Eulogy.
Thank you.
Thank you for your life and your work.
For Jazz, for Paradise, and for Home.
God Help the Child!
I'm so grateful.

My favorite elder is now an ancestor.
All Praises be!

Rest In Peace Queen Mother
Toni Morrison.

I can't believe it!

August 6, 2019

Sometimes we need every day reminders to let shit go.

I sure as hell do.

I'm often triggered by past trauma, but I'm healing! I actually realized recently that I'm holding on to a lot of trauma from college, attending a PWI, and all the fuck shit that went along with that—trauma bonding and unhealthy relationships and associations. Even to the point where I've been feeling regretful about having even attended college at all, and falling into the trap of student debt. I literally feel like I was tricked.

After college I did a lot of self-education and independent study and learned more than I did in all my years of learning.

My ancestors reminded me that they were self-taught.
We can learn and grow without creating debt.

You're not stuck.

Think new thoughts.

August 10, 2019

What is college?

And what did I learn that could have possibly cost $83,000 plus, with apparently almost $4,000 that I still owe the university. Incurring $1300 in interest every couple months.

That's nothing compared to other graduates and degree holders.

Although I still have never seen or held my degree or my official undergraduate collegiate transcripts.

Did college even happen?
Did I go through a "slaving" process?
Within a PWI—yes.
Within my Black affiliations on a predominately white campus—yes.

Moving to DC really woke me up.

We are raised to continue the slave-like mentality of the people before us and around us simply by being Black and low-income.

It's much easier to live a life fitting into the system of racism and white supremacy than it is to freely exist alongside it. Freedom fighters die, they are jailed, they are silenced in the most horrific ways. We're made to think we're crazy or that we deserve these conditions. The work we do should afford us the same lifestyle as them, if not, better.

Full Moon | August 17, 2019

Blessings.

I wish profound love and abundance to my family and friends—who love and support me. My ancestors for continuously having my back and providing me with the tools I need to be great.

For the full moon, I've been getting more in tune with my tarot deck. For the full moon, I called on Spirit to show me what I need to release. And I pulled the *Queen of Swords.* Which symbolizes an independent woman and single parents/moms.

It's interesting because I never thought spirit would ask me/ show me / reveal that I release this. I was raised to be an independent, single, woman. But no woman is truly a single mom. And those who are "single" suffer and their children suffer too. Maybe it's time we redefine what it means to be a single mother.

[Write whatever you need to release on a sheet of paper, and burn the paper]

Yesterday, on the third night of the full moon, I made a powerful release of what no longer serves me.

So it shall be done.

Melanie Julion

A name that is mine but no longer feels like mine. It feels like an idea of a person my parents tried to create, either knowingly or unknowingly. A person who lived in fear of the past and of repeating cycles and experiences of my ancestors and parents.

We must make our own path even if that means starting a whole new path so theres no way we'll be able to go back to hold habits, old thoughts, and experiences.

I am not Melanie Julion.

I am the spirit that resides within the body of a person called Melanie.

I am the color yellow.
I am a Black community gathering.
I am children learning.
I am women playing, praying, and slaying.
I am the unwavering elder.
I am abundance made manifest.
I am an old bookstore.
With free knowledge.
I am good pussy on a Friday night.
I am sleeping in on Saturdays and easy,
like brunch on Sunday morning.
I am the Divine.
I am light.
Mommy.
I am love.
I am truth.

I am justice.
I am a good book that never really ends.
I am a sesh.
I am cannabis.
I am.
I am not my parent's expectations.
I am not what my family thinks.
I am not who they think I am.
I am the light that brings out all darkness.
I am not your religion.
I am not your church.
I am the charm that your great-grandma kept and
the stones she held in her breast.
I am a woman of profound glory.
I am a woman.
I am a woman.
I am not your definition.
I am mine.
I am mine.
I belong to me.

I am Like
Water for
Chocolate City.

August 23, 2019

I've been on a journey learning about tarot and I am truly thankful to god, the Creator of the Universe, Spirit, my ancestors, and guides who have allowed me the opportunity to journey into my spirit and the spirit of the world

I've been reflecting on the 5 cards I pulled for the week:

Strength- The "Strong Black Woman" card

Page of Cups- "Message from/with young person

X of Swords- Welcome/Celebrated dying of former Self

V of Pentacles- Fear of poverty, financially poor, fear of losing security of home, sadness over loss (look up, practice gratitude)

Page of Wands- Good news, Communication, writer
Me in Africa

These cards revealed to me where I am in my journey. I am no doubt a strong woman who has tamed many wild animals with purity and compassion—in tune with the infinite. Fertile, listening to the meaning and messages of children and birth. Many parts of me have died and my current self no longer serves me. So, I release it. Proudly and bravely. I've suffered financially but have always been rich, whether I looked up to appreciated the beauty of my surroundings or not… I've connected and found safety and love and security in those who have been in similar emotional and financial places. The coldest of places—Chicago. And I used my intuition and wisdom to be where I am today. Now that I have my tribe, we can continue on our journey to know and see spirit—our homeland.

Let's get out of our cages.

And fly.

The caged bird
is free.

Free
Free
Free.

This week, all the cards that I've pulled and Messiah has pulled for me
(page of cups) show that we'll be moving spiritually moving forward and
physically moving into a new home within the next few months or so.

The curse is over.
The curse is broken.

Now we open our arms and
receive all that the universe has in store for us.

Our home.
Our land.
Our herbs.
Our food.

August 24, 2019

The *X of Swords* finally hit me. Literally laying here with swords in my back. My family has betrayed me in so many ways. I feel so heart broken. Then I realized I've always been the broken-hearted girl, the one crying over family problems, secrets, and hurt feelings. I've broken the curses. I am no longer a part of them.

Malcolm reminded me yesterday that I am almost 30, with no job, and two kids to take care of. He shamed me. I bet he slept better last night. Muhammed is so ashamed of me, it's just easier for him to never call. HH is too embarrassed. Sex before marriage. Baby out of wedlock. Not just one, but two. And I know the three of them think I deserve heartache and abuse. Muhammed has never said anything like, "Make sure Jackson does this, this, and this…make sure he treats you like this and never does this or that." He, nor HH, has never told me that I'm beautiful and that I deserve the world. They have never protected me. Never gave a fuck.

Patra only gives a fuck when it's something in it for her or something for her to talk about so she'll have the upper hand.

My mom couldn't give a fuck less about me and my babies. She's been everywhere but here to see me and her grandchildren at the very least.

I remember when I gave birth to Mars and she promised she was coming out here to help—"I'm not coming out there for you. I don't care about you. I'm coming to see my grandchildren—this is not about you," she told me. And still hasn't shown up.

This is the blood I come from.

These motherfuckers must hate me. They've literally made my life a living hell since I was a child. I can literally make a list of all the swords in my back from the people I thought supported me. But no, I won't! People only support you when it's convenient.

288

I will live the life I am destined to live and I will leave them all behind.

It's been five years since I moved to the east coast and not a damn soul has come out here with the purest of intentions of seeing how I am doing.

Red Flag!

No Family vacations? *Red Flag*
No phone call for the boys? *Red flag*
No gifts on the boys birthday? *Red Flag*
Malcolm didn't call you on your birthday
HH didn't even call you on Mother's Day
Did Muhammed?
These are the men I've attracted in my life?
And Jackson?
All the fucking red flags.

I am no longer focused on this life.
I am no longer setting up a life to live in this country.
My mind is on Africa.
I am on a mission.
I am not of here
and deserve much more
than this life can ever provide.

My children deserve more
and I will give them another life
in a better country.
In Ghana.

We are moving!

I released old clothes
and old energy,
old fears, habits,
and thoughts
that did not serve me.

I am anew.
It is okay to be who I've always dreamed of being.
I welcome complete security in my wealth, satisfaction, and love in my
home.
I am deserving.

I am abundant.
I am in tune.
I am melanin.
I am The Cannabis Doula.
I am a revolutionary mama.
I am peace.

I pulled "The Fool" card to release
and forgive myself for my foolish past.
I am grateful for my journey.

September 2, 2019

Leaves are changing from green to yellow and falling quickly to the ground. Although the heat and humidity of August in DC still lingers around like it's still mid-summer.

This summer was a quick one.

It was just spring when the surgeons at Johns Hopkins diagnosed me with thyroid cancer. I've managed to avoid surgery. Now it's the fall, and I'm starting to wonder about not just my physical health, but the emotional trauma and underlying, untreated mental illness that may be contributing to this cancer. I know it's my throat chakra and I know what needs to be said in order to release this blockage.

Today I pulled the *III of Swords* and I immediately knew:

My heart was broken, many, many times in my girlhood and I have yet to heal and release. But I release it now. *Here.*

My parents, who failed to teach me how to love, who failed to provide a safe, clean home with balanced healthy meals, who failed to provide us with adequate medical and dental care and mental health care, who never hugged us and said "I love you."

I release the anger I have for my parents for not parenting me the way I feel like my siblings and I deserved to be parented.

I release my parents for not being good grandparents to my babies.

I release my parents for asking "what did you do?" when I told them Jackson put his hands on me.

I release my parents for telling my business and exaggerating the truth.

I release my parents for not properly raising or caring for my little brother.

I release my parents for shaming us.

I release my parents for their toxicity and desire to conform.

I release Muhammed for not attending any of my graduations and for not acknowledging my babies.

I release any feelings of shame I may have felt during my pregnancy with messiah because of the lack of love and support I received.

I release the feelings of jealousy I feel of healthy mother-daughter and father-daughter relationships

I release the tensions in my shoulders.

I inhale peace and exhale everything that has never served me.

I release my parents for reading my journals, shaming, and punishing me for my thoughts and feelings. It did irreparable damage to my confidence and self-expression. It is released.

I release my parents for using God to justify their poor parenting choices, financial decisions, and overall lack of care, empathy, and miseducation.

I release my parents for being poor mentors and spiritual gods and surrounding me with poor examples of love, happiness, peace, and abundance.

I release my parents for making me go to college and acquiring over $85,000 in debt just to make them look good.

I release my parents for never taking us (me) out of the country or on any vacation.

I release my parents for shaming my brother for his love of Africa and when he received his African name.

I release my dad for whoopin' us with snake-skin belts and collecting them for the purpose of whoopin' us.

I release HH for recording our phone calls.

I release my mom for staying even after we told her he was recording phone calls.

I release the feeling of guilt for never telling on HH for recording our phone calls and opening/hiding our mail.

I release the shame and anger I felt because Muhammed didn't protect my mom. I release the toxic idea that it was his job, or responsibility.

I release the feeling that my brothers were weak because they didn't stop HH's abuse.

I release negative feelings I have toward Muhammed for still being cool with HH and supporting his dysfunctional behavior.

I forgive my mom for still fucking HH after he had her car stolen.

I forgive my mom for her ignorance of her own sexual power and for teaching me to ignore my sexual power.

I forgive my parents for shaming me when Mitchell died, when Kristina died, and not even caring or acknowledging Jasmine's death.

I release the feeling of guilt I have for pledging, and hazing, and submitting to being hazed.

I release the slave mentality that my parents passed down to me.

I release the feeling and learned behavior of poverty, loss, and struggle.

I release being poor and broke.

I release poor health, that my parents have passed down.

I release hatred I feel for not having inherited land, property, or trade from my family.

I release post-traumatic slave syndrome.

I release my parents for shaming me as a girl about my body, hair, and clothes—instead of teaching.

I release my dad for constantly calling my mom a hoe and bitch and for thinking the same about me and my sister.

I release the loneliness I felt throughout childhood and seeking sexual fulfillment in place of being lonely.

I release moments of nonconsensual sex and rape that I experienced in college, and after.

I release the guilt of sleeping with men who were involved with other women.

I release the false sense of freedom I felt from making irresponsible, hurtful decisions.

I release the negative energy I carry from past relationships, and old flames.

I release feelings of lack of self-worth, self-pity, and self-victimization.

I release feelings of lack and poverty.

I release the poor-man mentality and open my arms proudly to receive full abundance, love, light, and peace from spirit.

I welcome land, property, money, gems, crystals, books, herbs, knowledge from my ancestors, Spirit, and guides.

The day after the new moon, a butterfly landed on me.

So shall it be.

Crystals & Cannabis
Throat Chakra Healing

Blue Obsidian
Angelite / Anhydrite
Lapis Lazuli
Turquenite
Amethyst
Blue sandstone
Tiger's Eye
Blue Lace Agate
Flourite
Rose Quartz
Snowflake Obsidian
Green Adventurine
Aquamarine
Citrine
Sodalite
Carnelian
Clear Quartz
Black Onyx

The ocean, water, sand, healing, clarity, truth, flow, cleanse, release.

September 9, 2019

How unsettling it is to realize just how emotionally, mentally, and spiritually enslaving Christianity is to the Black body.

I had no idea the vastness of creation, no idea of the true beauty of the universe.

I offer my deepest gratitude to the earth, our mother.

I recognize my place in the universe, I am.

I am the true universe in its greatest expression as a spiritual being in an earthly realm manifested as a Black girl from the south side of Chicago.

In my lower form, I experienced all the things that Melanie experienced in human form—suffering. I allowed people, institutions, corporations and the government to deposit information in me with the belief that I was receiving "knowledge."

It took me a full five years to unlearn and relearn all the information I received in high school and college.

Neither setting taught me about me, my Self, or my people. Only you can do that. (It's no one's job to teach our children our history, but us.) I'm still learning and everyday I'm learning that I still have more to learn and I pray that learning takes me across the ocean, back to the homeland.

Sometimes our families will fail (to teach, to show) us.
Our friends will abandon us. And society will silence you. But stand whole and speak truth anyway. Be Black anyway. Be. Anyway. Woman-ish. Woman. Un-Woman. Non-Woman. Womanly.
Be Every Woman.

Go back + seek it. Love your babies. Learn to love and trust Black men, everyday all over again. Love is a continual doing. A continual being.

Forgive yourself for what you did or didn't do when you were broken, chained, and miseducated, neglected and unloved.

You've been cold your whole life.
It's okay to expect the sun.
Turn in the direction of the sun, you sunflower.
Let it rebirth in you a love and warmth that will last for generations.

Keep the bees.
Grow the weed.
And love,
love,
love,
love.

"I'm every woman
It's all in me.
Anything
You want done, baby.
I do it naturally.

-Nippy

Full Moon | September 13, 2019

What have I created and manifested since the new moon:
VII of Swords

Where am I now?
Page of Wands

What is coming into my conscious awareness?
Strength

What is no longer serving me?
X of Cups

How can I release / let go of these energies?
Knight of Pentacles

What additional resources are available to me as I release and let go?
Knight of Swords

Clarify the *X of Cups*

    Past- *VII of Cups*
    Present- *II of Cups*
    Future- *II of Wands*

My doctors don't support
using medical cannabis for thyroid cancer.

I am confident
and knowledgeable
and have the ability to heal myself;
whether people believe me / support me or not.
I am a healer.

I can be,
I will be,
I am
a wonderful,
loving
and peaceful
mother
and a powerful,
wealthy,
successful entrepreneur.

September 17, 2019

I found an ENT doctor who is somewhat open to learning about cannabis as a therapeutic treatment to heal my thyroid and he's Black.

Thank you ancestors.

I'm still trying to speak my truth and be bold and confident with who I am. I'll admit, its extremely challenging.

I'm thankful for Lapis Lazuli and Blue Lace Agate for the healing energy.

An overactive thyroid, and an underactive thyroid, both have negative effects and I feel like I'm experiencing both. But more so, let me just be honest.

No other female mammal depends on a male to feed herself and her young, or to house her. No wonder I'm sick and I feel like I can't speak. I'm not living in harmony with the wild woman, the inner woman that is often buried or dies when a woman marries. A single mama is a powerful one.

Today Jackson said to me, "Stop talking to me like you're the only woman in the world." Yesterday, I had to leave the house when he got mad because I don't eat as much as I used to since becoming vegan.

It's true. I don't eat as much and the thought of toxins and GMOs, fluoride water, heavy metals present in most food is enough to have me fasting intermittently everyday. He was literally screaming and cursing and two days prior had the audacity to text HH what I told him the doctor had said.

Whole time I've been asking for "signs." Loud and clear. I get it now. I'm ready.

Jackson and I need time and space and I recognize that. He wants me at home and working toward his dream, not mine. As long as I'm watching his kids, he's okay. He's not ready to support me and the boys the way we need and I do not deserve to struggle. He could be cheating. He could be lying, gas lighting, and could be blinded thinking it's love and protection.

He has a low emotional IQ. Yesterday I told him he was emotionally-retarded and as harsh as that may sound I think it accurately describes his inability to understand my emotions and respond with appropriate emotions. There is no reason why a 30-year-old man responds to my being sick with anger, my healing with anger. I've tried my best to help him live his dream but I can't do it for him; even if he thinks I owe him for being at work for 8 hours a day. He literally thinks I owe him.

He only just started putting the boys to sleep last week. What the fuck is this? How did I think someone with no dad in his life could grow up to be a better dad? With no support and no resources! I refuse to raise another generation of angry, emotionally unintelligent Black male children.

I don't need anymore signs.

I am ready to continue my journey with two little boys in tow.
I have so much love to give and I know I am worthy of much more than I've been settling for.

Full Moon | October 13, 2019

I have a three year old now.
And a 1 ½ year old.
I love them more than I love myself and because I love them so much I
think they deserve to have a happy, healthy mother.

In celebrating Messiah's 3 years of life—I also celebrated my first three
years as a mom—and went out for the first time without one or both of
them. We didn't do anything special, other than what Jackson wanted
to do. I've been doing what he wanted to do the entirety of our relationship. I settled for far less than what I deserve and I know now that
I can never be happy in this relationship and for most of this time, my
happiness relied on him being happy.

This full moon has really awakened me to how I've given my power
away and have been repeating the same cycle for years.

I feared being alone.
I feared what people would think of me as a single mom.
But I deserve more.
I can see me dying if I don't properly heal from the emotional pain and
trauma I've experienced.

If I continue to be silent about my pain— they will kill me and say I
enjoyed it. Word to Zora Neale Hurston.

Things I need to release:

Domestic violence in the form of partner to partner violence, parent to
child violence, emotional abuse and neglect, psychological abuse, gas-
lighting, financial abuse, poverty, poor education, religious abuse, with-
holding information, secrets, lies, deception, manipulation, and narcis-
sism.

I release it all.

It has never served me.
I release it from impacting my future.

People I need to release:

I release all narcissistic people, friends, lovers, and family who continue to inflict pain on to me and others. I release Jackson. I release my mom. I release HH. I release manipulators, liars, and people who intend to do me harm. I release Jackson's mother. I release people who speak ill of me behind my back. I release "friends" who don't see me as worthy of care and support.

I release everyone with whom I've ever formed a bond/ relationship/ sisterhood from trauma, pain, or despair.

I release every one of my sorority sisters and the toxic relationships that were formed and rooted in the trauma of hazing. They know their names.

People I need to forgive:

I forgive Jackson for treating me the only way he knows how. I forgive myself for falling for his toxicity. I forgive him for being abusive and for choosing not to get support.

I forgive my parents for doing the best they could.

I forgive my family for not caring enough to help me.

I forgive HH for making us homeless.

I forgive myself for accepting the energy people have given me all these years.

People/ Things I need to be grateful for:

I'm grateful for my children.

I'm grateful for my birth experiences.

304

I'm grateful for Jen.

I'm grateful for Kim; for telling me they love me yesterday.

I'm grateful for genuine sisterhood.

I'm grateful for cannabis.

I'm grateful that I've been able to be with my children everyday.

I welcome love, support, wealth, and health in place of all that I have released.

Asé

Sun _____

Rising _____

Moon_____

Astrological Birth Data

Planet	Sign
Sun	_____
Moon	_____
Mercury	_____
Venus	_____
Mars	_____
Jupiter	_____
Saturn	_____
Uranus	_____
Pluto	_____
North Node	_____
Neptune	_____

Understanding your astrological birth chart can help us to navigate various transitions throughout our lives and make decisions that are better in tune with the universe.

October 25, 2019

The teachers are striking in Chicago and everybody's worried about the children.

The teachers want better conditions, librarians, nurses, aids, and smaller class sizes. Of course, higher pay. Rightfully so.

I express sincere gratitude to the Chicago Public Schools and the Chicago's Teacher Union. If I were in Chicago, I'd probably be out in protest with them in complete solidarity.

Thing is, we need a whole restructuring of the educational system in Chicago. Budgets have been getting cut continuously, repeatedly, for years. More funding is spent on police officers in schools than on counselors, nurses, and librarians. Our schools are prisons (but melanated people aren't shooting up schools!)

Like at Hubbard, just recently as 2015 when I went to visit a former teacher. They had removed all the mirrors in the girls bathroom (of course, no soap, and no paper towels) and when I inquired about it, he said the same thing teachers and security guards were saying about students using the girls bathroom back when I was a student there—"its too much of a distraction."

I wish I could expound on what that means, but I still don't know if it's distracting to the teachers or to the students. I remember the inappropriate comments teachers would make about students. It really should be the students who ought to be on strike. I know more students than I can name who've suffered abuse from teachers within the Chicago Public School system, especially at Hubbard High School.

The CPS system is doing what it was designed to do. They close schools, fire teachers, cut budgets, cut resources, increase test score requirements, require longer school days, teachers demand more pay, students fail to meet standards, district blames teachers, deny pay increase and resources, teachers blame parents, students, and the districts. Teachers strike.

District will respond by completely wiping out the CPS system bringing in private corporations to introduce their charter schools. Giving complete control of our children's education to strangers and perhaps people will see this as a win. But is it? Who's teaching your children?

I'll tell you who I see at the library every day, every week, teaching, playing, and reading to white children:
-their parents
-their grandparents
-their nannies/sitters (white, Black, Latina, Indian, African, and women of all ethnicities)

Who's watching your baby while you are taking care of someone else's and why do we prioritize the needs of white children and white families over the needs of our own children and community?

Who's teaching Black children?

A lot of educators who don't like their jobs. Educators who are abused by student's misplaced anger (students should have been on strike long time ago). Teachers who are underpaid and overworked cannot possibly have the creative energy to passionately influence a classroom of nearly 35 intelligent Black minds.

It takes a village.

I had a lot of "friends" who were teachers in CPS who in 2015 when Black youth across the country were quitting their jobs, missing school to take to the streets in protest of the unjust killing of Mike Brown (and others), it was these teachers who were saying, "no—I'd never do no shit like that. I'd never risk my salary to protest no shit that's not gone change." Several teachers. Shamed our youth. The educators of our community, not standing alongside and fighting with the very youth that they teach everyday, who were only demanding not to be killed; who were only demanding equal protection.

Our schools are over-policed. Our policies are abusive to students and teachers contribute to the abusive conditions. They accept it. I think that Black students deserve better.

When you leave Chicago (or DC or Baltimore) and live in such a county as Montgomery County, Maryland you realize the CPS students don't have nearly the percentage of the resources these students have.

They just opened and IB World School here in Silver Spring!

These white schools would not dear have metal detectors to such degree as a Black/Latino schools, nor would they have a full time officer on duty—with his own office, like at Hubbard.

What is it to even be considered a graduate of such a school in such a neighborhood? It came out not too long ago that teachers from Hubbard High School were being investigated for sexual misconduct with students.

We all knew.
Why didn't we say anything? Did we think it was normal for teachers to flirt? Did we think it was normal for security guards to look at our asses?
Did we think it was cool for teachers to fuck the football players?
What are these schools really?
What did they teach us?
I was taught that women were to be seen and not heard.
I was taught that my looks were distracting.
I was taught to keep quiet about abuse.
I was taught to just say fuck it.
Whatever is done in the dark will come to light eventually.
Malcolm X said, "only a fool would let his enemy educate his children."

I release the guilt of not having spoken up against the injustices that we faced as students.

Like when they fired our Black cheerleading coach and replaced her with a white teacher without any warning. They fired our cheerleading coach because they thought our dances were too provocative. They policed our bodies. I release it.

A former teacher told me that my high school boyfriend had sex with a teacher, Ms. Certa, when we were in high school. When I started to curse him, he stopped me. "They were kids. They were boys. She was an adult."

Why didn't we know that?
Why didn't they tell us that then?
That we were children.

It didn't feel like we were children.

When I heard Ms. Certa was pregnant by another football player, I didn't think of it as inappropriate until I realized he was a child and she was his teacher.

They were abusing us.

They were teaching us not to love ourselves and that if someone was sexually attracted to you, it was your obligation to fulfill their desires.

What other forms of abuse have teachers unknowingly taught to Black students to keep us inferior?

Do they even know that they are a part of the very system they detest?

That, even on strike, they are working with teachers who actively suspend more Black students than white ones?

Are all the teachers protesting? Someone has to know something.

Aside from the teachers striking in Chicago—I woke up to some memories. Memories of wearing all white, chanting, with other Black women and girls wearing white. "Saint Peter Claver, Pray for us." We'd say repeatedly, over and over again.

There'd be other Black men wearing funny hats leading us in these prayers. Some we knew from our church, but most of these people we'd never seen before. But our parents had me and my sister attending these meetings of these junior daughters of the Knights of Peter Claver.

and I woke up like...

Who the FUCK is Peter Claver?!

"Saint" Peter Claver was a catholic priest in South America who dedicated his life to converting enslaved African people to Christianity. Most White people found it repulsive but also worthy of sainthood because according to the catholic church, African people were, "the least of these."

He was not all light (or a saint at all.) He'd severely beat slaves for dancing and drumming. The "slave of slaves" owned slaves himself. He would greet arriving slave ships of African people who thought there were going to be eaten alive. A frightened people. Their lives destroyed and their spiritual practices—stripped from them, and replaced with Christianity. I weep for my ancestors. And "Saint" Sabina.

November 2, 2019

The teachers' strike ended. 10 days.
I know a lot of teachers and coaches in the Chicago Public Schools and surrounding areas who go above and beyond for their students and know to show humility and grace, and respect for their parents. I also know teachers who get on social media and talk straight trash about their classrooms and schools, parents and students. I've seen teachers work other jobs just to further support their students. Being a teacher is a lifestyle, not a job and a lot of people unfortunately take advantage of their responsibility as an educator. They conform and become complicit in a system that is destroying our communities (literally!) across the country. Why are we still participating in the school to prison pipeline? Why are we still teaching in and sending our children to schools that mirror detention centers?

John Witherspoon died a few days ago.

It was crazy but I was hoping through his character on Black Jesus, he'd somehow wake people up. God is in you! You are a God. Our lives as Black people in this country will always mirror the life of Jesus Christ, because we are the Chosen People. We are magic.. We are alchemists. We heal, we build, we grow. We speak truth, because we know. Our ancestors knew.

Pick up the torch.

Talk to the elders.

Love the children.
And make mad love.

Seek inward. You have everything you need. You are worth more than gold.

I am melanin. I am melanin. I am melanin. I am melanin. I am melanin. I am melanin. I am loved. I am whole.. I am protected. I am evolving.

Mercury is in retrograde. A new moon is among us.

I turned down another job in cannabis, this time an Assistant Manager position at a local dispensary. I felt like $57,000 wasn't enough. I tried to negotiate $3,000 additional. I feel really strongly that I'm worth at least 60k a year. I have two babies. I'll walk away with my worth on this one—although I'm kicking myself. How you let 57k slip?

I am worth more.
I am worth more.
I am worth more.

I pray for my health and healing.
I pray that my ancestors and spirit guides cover me and lead me with a clear path to my wealth and abundance.

I pray that my voice is strong and my heart is light. I pray that my message is received in light and in love.

I pray you hear me.
God is the single manifestation of love; of you!
God, The Creator, The Universe, and you are all one.
You are the ebb and flow of all the Earth.

You are the good and bad.
The light and the dark.
The whole and the broken.
The rich and the poor.
The Black
And the white.

I don't know why we're here or if we'll ever get reparations, the land or the resources.

But I do know that we're all one people, one body, like Osiris, scattered all around the world. And the only way to be whole, to be free, in this lifetime, is to pick up the pieces and put them back together again.

Like shopping at a foreign grocery,

Except instead of expecting foreign owners to help you—remember, their job is to make a profit—look to your sister, look to your brother, look to your mom, if you can.

If not, that's okay.

We all gone eat.

This week an Elder told me to tell you:

1. Elijah Cummings died. Look into that.
2. Rosa Parks death anniversary was the other day. Look—raise hell in any way you can.
3. Sit down and listen.
4. The Amish grow food in Pennsylvania and they bring the produce down to the Dutch Farmers Market in Laurel, MD. It's open every weekend. And they sale mostly to the Jewish people. Fresher than anything you'll get at this grocery store. (He used to go every weekend until he said they damaged his car so he had to stop going.)

Medical Cannabis Therapeutics: Cancer

Mon, Nov 4, 2019, 12:48 PM

Greetings Dr. Mathers & Dr. Thompson:

I've included links to research studies and various articles and videos related to medical cannabis, Thyroid disorders, and cancer. I look forward to hearing your thoughts and concerns. With the guidance of my certifying physician, Stephanie James, I am currently a medical cannabis patient and I'm incorporating various forms of cannabis into my daily wellness routines. My goal is to shrink the nodules on and around my Thyroid, to kill and repair any cancerous cells, and manage all other symptoms with cannabis, various herbs and natural remedies, including diet and lifestyle changes.

Thank you for your patience and consideration.

All the best,
Melanie

Medical Marijuana for Thyroid Cancer
   https://www.marijuanadoctors.com/conditions/thyroid-cancer/

Clinical Significance of Cannabinoid Receptors CB1 and CB2 Expression in Human Malignant and Benign Thyroid Lesions
   https://www.ncbi.nlm.nih.gov/pmc/articles/PMC4619873/

THE IMPACT CBD HAS ON THYROID DISEASE/DISORDER
   https://infinitecbd.com/the-impact-cbd-has-on-thyroid-disease-disorder/

Prospective Analysis of Safety and Efficacy of Medical Cannabis in Large Unselected Population of Patients with Cancer
   https://www.sativaisticated.com/wp-content/uploads/2018/05/

Prospective-analysis-of-safety-and-efficacy-of-medical-canna-
bis-in-large-unselected-population-of-patients-with-cancer-Medi-
cal-Cannabis-Medical-Marijuana-Study-for-Treating-Cancer.pdf

Endocannabinoids and the Endocrine System in Health and Disease
https://www.ncbi.nlm.nih.gov/pmc/articles/PMC6813821/

RSO Cannabis Oil
https://cannabiscure.info/rso-cannabis-oil/

CBD for Thyroid Disorders
https://nordicoil.com/wiki/cbd-for-thyroid-disorders/

**Effect of Marijuana Use on Thyroid Function and Autoimmu-
nity**
https://www.liebertpub.com/doi/full/10.1089/
thy.2016.0197?url_ver=Z39.88-2003&rfr_
id=ori%3Arid%3Acrossref.org&rfr_dat=cr_pub%3Dpubmed&

Videos:

Run For The Cure - The Rick Simpson Story
https://m.youtube.com/watch?v=zDJX7GqsQoA

Cannabis Cures Cancer
https://m.youtube.com/watch?v=NAnjvC7rsE8

Other Resources:

Cannabis Education, resources, and more
https://www.green-flower.com

Rick Simpson & RSO Dosage Information
https://phoenixtears.ca/dosage-information/

November 20, 2019

My ancestors have guided me here.
Asé.
My ancestors have protected me and have covered me!
All praises be!
To thy ancestors.

Grams carried me.
My grandma has carried me.
My mom has carried me.
Today she texted me and said
She misses my skin.
I miss hers, too.

All praises be
To the women who raised me.
My mom, her chocolate brown skin
Will forever be etched in my mind
As the standard of beauty.
You mean to me
What the sun means to the sky.
Asé Ajé Asé

We look to our mothers—yes.
But we must also look to our community.
To heal and to grow
To reconnect—as one.
The ones who remember.

I speak truth. I am love.
I walk in my power.
I am melanin.
I am melanie.
I am melanin ajé

I am here to educate and serve.
To teach .
With cannabis.
To heal
women and children
of the Diaspora.

Cannabis is our birthright.

In 2020, I welcome financial, spiritual, and physical abundance. Like Water for Chocolate City will be manifested in spring, a beautiful representation of Black girlhood. I will impact the lives of women and girls through Melanin & Books— The Black Girl Monarch Collective (BGM), I will support Black birthing families through Happy Brown Baby and educate and provide exceptional care through The Cannabis Doula. I will bring cannabis use mainstream to support Black birthing women across the Diaspora. All the positivity and love will be attracted to me.

I welcome all abundance, joy, and light.

Melanin Ajé Seshat
is the manifestation of my highest self.

She is deeply intuitive.
And knowledgeable.
She is in tune with the ancestors and
Praised by the elders.

I love cannabis.
I love books.
I love writing, words and poetry.
I love Black culture, people, history.

I seek the love of mama Africa
I am a wanderer; lost at sea
My home is in Africa.
To Africa I will return.

I will be one of the wealthiest
Women in Africa.
I will be the wealthiest Black woman
cannabis entrepreneur.

I will reap a plentiful harvest
for many generations to come.

Plant-based diet
Daily Yoga
Pole fitness
  -conditioning
  -classes
  -home pole

Tarot
  -daily, reading for self and others

Journal daily
Sacred Retreats

Full expression of true self; highest self.
True communication of needs of self.
Self-Love mastery.
Reconnect with Africa.

*"Lies become history when
everyday people don't tell their truth."*

-Yeye Luisah Teish

Dreamworks Masterclass

Treasure from a Dead Man's Chest, Jambalaya p. 158

Dreams
- Improve alpha state to remember dreams
- Ancestors communicate through dreams
- Dream, wake up, write it down, drink water, write, lay down
- Inquire with others about their dreams

Prophetic Dreaming
- Keep track of dreaming
- Look out for those with similar dreams

How to Dispel a Hant, Jambalaya pg. 181-191

I am grateful for the healing.
I am grateful for the shifts.
My highest inner self being manifested outward.
This winter solstice has provided so much insight
and confirmation from the
ancestors.

I realized the toxicity of our relationships
usually start at the root…the foundation.
Jackson and I cannot get married.
The whole foundation of our relationship was started
on him still liking his ex-girlfriend.

I've been living in her shadow—for five years.
We had two children.
I found some old pictures of them together;
pics he said he had deleted.
He hid them in another folder.
He said he still had feelings for her.
I was pregnant with Messiah when I
asked him to delete the pics.
Why do you still have these?
He said he wanted to show them to Messiah
When he got older.
He said he deleted them.
He kept them in a hidden dropbox for five years.

Our whole relationship was built on him still liking,
thinking about, getting over his ex.
So how much time has he really been with me?
He said he was in love with me.
I was pregnant with Messiah.
He still liked his ex.
There were red flags. I largely ignored them.

He doesn't adore me.
Or admire me.
He supports me only far enough
so he doesn't look like a bad guy.

And when he does look like a bad guy—He says he's not perfect and I should go find my dream man. He always tells me to leave. Literally since the beginning of our relationship, he's threatened to kick me out or suggested I leave. His mom told my parents that I should put him on child support.

Throws red flag

Like the ancestors say— and like Yeye Teish reminded me, all roads lead back to center. No matter what decision I make between DC and California, between me and Jackson— all will lead to a more centered/balanced existence.

I am grateful for a beautiful life in California.
I'm grateful for my ability to start a new chapter of my life.
Focused on healing and growth.

Physically, I am grateful for the strength and endurance that pole fitness, dance, and yoga will give me and I am grateful for every opportunity that the universe is providing to manifest my greatest physical self.

Financially, I am grateful for the abundance of wealth that a full time dispensary job will provide and opportunities to network and learn to build generational wealth through hemp and cannabis. I attract all cannabis networks and job opportunities in the San Francisco Bay Area, Berkeley, Oakland. I will make an impact in the cannabis industry.

I am grateful for the scholarship opportunities that I continue to receive as gifts to and from my ancestors.

I am grateful that my cannabis events have been successful and I will continue to attract Black spirits back to our natural plant medicine— cannabis.

I am grateful for the lives that will save and birth as a midwife concentrating on cannabis therapeutics for pregnancy, childbirth, and postpartum.

I am a legend.
I am grateful for my ancestral knowledge to seek truth in using cannabis to safely heal our community from birth to death. Supporting life's transitions as cannabis always has. Asé.

I am grateful for the home that I am building and the village I'm continuing to manifest.

My intention is to move to the Oakland Bay Area by securing a $65,000 salary annually. I will attend the Master's Entry nursing programs at the University of California- San Francisco for a Certified Nurse Midwife - Women's Health Nurse Practitioner credential preparing me to for the work of my ancestors all over the world, especially in Africa. All for mama Africa. I have my gardens, my beautiful estate, and all mama's babies.

I am like water and I
Pray I continue with the ebb and flow
Sometimes crushing
Other times
Still
Silent
Wearing
Dripping
Leaking
Melting
Like chocolate
Between the fingers
And mouths of two lovers
Or a toddler
Thirsty for more.
I give
Offerings
To Oshun.
Like honey
to heal.

Egyptian Zodiac: _____

    Traits: _____

    Lucky colors: _____

    Characteristics: _____

    _____

    _____

African Zodiac
(African Geomancy): _____

    Favorable day: _____

    Sensitive body parts: _____

    Sense: _____

    Element: _____

    Success months: _____

    Key Characteristics: _____

    _____

December 24, 2019

I am grateful for the wealth
that I am receiving for The Cannabis Doula,
Happy Brown Baby and Melanin & Books.

I am open and ready
to receive great financial wealth, property/real estate.

I am grateful for security, love, and protection.

I have all the wealth and abundance that I am worthy.

I am worthy.

I am thankful.

I am rich.

I am healthy.

I am wealthy.

I am wise.

December 25, 2019

"Water that stays still eventually stagnates and becomes toxic."

The words jumped out at me.
Loudly.

As a reminder that it's time for me to keep flow.

1.   Current position —*III of wands*
2.   What you expect out of life right now— *Temperance*
3.   What you do not expect, a surprise —*VIII of Wands*
4.   Immediate Future — *X of Swords*
5.   Long Term Future (coming year) —*IV of Swords*

Thank you.

I've been nervous to pull cards because I knew what I'd see.
I know it will be a rough transition but it will be worth it.
I'm so grateful for this journey and I thank my ancestors for the money and abundance as I go to #Cali2020.

New Moon Solar Eclipse

May my vision board be made live in my reality in 2020.

All abundance and wealth is coming with the next full moon. My arms are open wide to receive all that I've asked for. I'm ready.

I'm thankful for the opportunity to teach outdoor play to children and families.

I can teach
a n y w h e r e !

I am thankful for the University of California for having an accelerated masters degree nursing program that will lead me to being a certified nurse midwife.

I am grateful for all the connections, resources, funding and support I am receiving for ALL of my work.

A future pole dancing nurse?

January 4, 2020

We made it to 2020.

I'm grateful to be present in this moment. True joy. I claim it all
All the sunshine, sunflowers.

The glow—in the darkest of winter. I feel aglow.
I see bees.
Honey flowing.
Watermelon dripping.
Cannabis smoking.
Love.
Babies and babies
And babies
Of love.
I have everything that I desire and even things I manifested as I write
this, as I breathe.

All my energy is manifested for my highest good. I pray for the knowledge to properly handle the money that I am receiving. I am wealthy.
And I am manifesting businesses, owning property, and doing what I
love everyday.

In 2020, I pray I make an impact that benefits the lives of women and
children all over the world. I pray The Cannabis Doula | Happy Brown
Baby flourishes in a miraculous way to our own brick and mortar.

Where we can teach and build.
I pray for all my travels in 2020.
I pray for my best recovery.
I pray for the completion of LW4CC.
I pray that everyone has the cannabis they need to be their best selves.
I pray for my highest Self.
I pray I do my best in articulating everything spirit has to teach and
uses me to do so.

I'm thankful for the lives I will touch in 2020
I am thankful for the millions of people who will buy my books.
I am grateful for truth.

January 8, 2020

Dear Jasmine,

I think I've finally summoned the courage to write to you.

Happy Birthday.
I miss you so much g.
I've been crying for two days.
I woke up at 12am on your birthday
And I knew exactly why.

I just want to thank you for being such an
amazing friend.
I did not deserve you.
Thank you for protecting me
With yo' tall ass!
I know now, after being diagnosed with cancer,
how things change
so quickly.
Your messages keep me going.
You always cheered for me.
I'll never get over this.
Maybe I'm not supposed to.
Maybe this was all part of
some universal plan to motivate
me to fight this cancer.
Naturally.
To be a better friend.
A better parent.

I lost an incredible friend.
We have so many memories
And each of them
involved you being so kind to me
at times when I was hurt, broken,

My lowest of low,
You were always there.
And when you needed me,
I was gone.

Was it by fate?
I would not have survived seeing you sick;
Worse than I am now.
Fucking chemo.
Cancer is a wake up call.
A reminder to be present, to heal, recover, and forgive;
To love, warmly.
Thank you for leaving behind
words for me to read
when I get sad.

You always had the best advice.
Thank you for reminding me
to live my dreams.

"Jasmine, come smoke!"
Man, I just wish I was there to
Get you to smoke.
Would've helped you eat,
At the very least,
You'd still be here
today.

I will never stop
fighting for you.

January 9, 2020

I welcome all abundance.
Of financial growth.
And prosperity.
I welcome healing.
I welcome joy.
The joy that comes
The morning after
The storm.
I welcome a new home.
And fulfillment.
I welcome peace.

Speak Life

I receive love, joy and truth.

I welcome growth and understanding.

Healing and Recovery.

Joy.

I have to start my own girls' group to honor Jasmine and Kristina. I have to find joy in my grief. Grieving is a life long thing. We have to find new ways to heal and cope with loss. Creatively. Joyfully. Fully.

I dance under the full moon
in celebration of what's to come.

I release all the heartache
and pain I had to
suffer in order to celebrate life.

I am limitless *(the limit does not exist!)*
I am healing.
I am recovering.
Restoring future generations
And I've already won

The *IX of Cups* reminds me
To be confident and unwavering— bold.
Here's what I've got—now pay me what I'm worth.

Let all the money and riches flow.
Like water.
Flood the place.

Remind me of my ancestor's wealth.
Grace me with their luxury.
I am grateful.
I sit on my throne in full
Abundance. Joy. Grace.

January 12, 2020

Turn poison (and pain) into medicine.

And I'm doing exactly that.
With a lot of spiritual herbal baths.
Reflection.
I'm also implementing other forms of self care into my life
Healing
Restoration
Celebration.

I can do this.
I was inspired by cheerleaders today.
I can never give up.
And can't even say it;
joke about it.

I have to change my thinking
And detox my body
       +   physical exercise
       +   lots of water
       +   therapy

I am learning to heal and healing.
I pray for peace within
as I release all that
no longer serves me...

and welcome the life that I've dreamed of...

(Pole dancing and maybe, cheerleading coach?!)

January 13, 2020

I am thankful for my ancestors;
the wise women who's stories
remind us
that
we are still
at war.

Delta Sigma Theta 107th Founders Day

I wonder what the founders
would think.

I wonder if Dorthy Irene Height
was thinking about how she would be president one day.
Sitting in her room manifesting
how she'd create the five-point
programmatic thrust.

I think about how I'll be president of Delta Sigma Theta...
One day—our focus will be on healing and restoration.

Can you imagine what would happen
if Delta was what I wanted it to be...

I wonder if Deltas with more money have a better chance of becoming
President...I already feel prepared.
In due time.

January 13, 2020

I welcome $ to heal and
treat all illness that may be
affecting my mind-body-spirit.

I wake up to gratitude.

I wake up full, light, and warm.

I wake up in love and peace.

I welcome $ for the sacred water retreat.

I welcome $ for an apartment.

I welcome $ for my self care,
the care of my babies and my community.

Sea salt lamp
Sound healing bowls
Exercise and pole
New clothes
Hair and glamour
Healthy food
Clean home
Crystals

January 15, 2020

I come from women.
Root women.
Strong women.
Never be dependent on a man.
They told me.
I thought learning to trust and love
Jackson meant that I had to completely
depend on him.
He wanted me to depend on him
To prove to himself,
His ego,
more than anything,
that he's a man and he can
take care of his family.
That he's dependable.
And he is,
to the best of his ability.
With what he can afford,
and handle.
It's stressful for him.
It's toxic.
Now so is he.
As are we.

Breaking the cycle is not never depending
or completely depending—
It's being *able* to depend on our men.

Choose a partner that you
are *able* to depend on,
Don't completely depend on them.
Or choose to never depend on them.

I have to be able to
Support myself and my dreams
And not completely depend
On the support from other people

Along the way.

I will continue to be disappointed.
But if I am establishing comfortable
boundaries where I am
able to depend on the people
in my circle
without being
completely dependent,
I can bring much joy into
my life.

I'm moving forward and welcome the transition
of being in my own place.
It will be great for me.
My health, happiness
and holistic well-being.

I'm excited to start pole.
Live lighter, released, restored
And welcome all the financial
Abundance I am due.

$ I am leading two early learning classes in the spring.
$ I am launching my holistic cannabis consumption: pregnancy, child-
birth, postpartum workshop.
$ I am teaching childbirth education.
$ I am preparing for midwifery school .
$ I am attending births as a HypnoDoula.
$ I am starting a homeschool coop and childcare academy.
$ I am creating cannabis and herb infused products.
$ I am learning real estate!

I am grateful for the path my ancestors have chosen for me.

I will be a midwife like Grams.
And I will go to nursing school
Because she was not able to.
I welcome me and my babies as
We welcome transitions.

January 17, 2020

Women,
We're taught as girls to
cling to men who can
love us
support us
and care for us,
especially financially.

Not only are we taught this,
we are often left with little options
in supporting ourselves
without relying on men.
Some women do this outright with no
shame—chase men with money, or
status
or worse, potential.
Other women do this secretly,
in quiet,
making sure he checks all the right boxes,
offering us a life we wouldn't be
able to give ourselves in
a patriarchal society.
And some women,
have so much of their own money, status,
and power,
that they want so very
little to do with and expect so much less
from men that their energy aligns enough to
repel a nothing ass man.

I welcome *that* type of energy into my spirit and
I will have nothing more to do
With these
vampires.

I am a great woman.
I am creative, beautiful, and empowered.
I expect the best quality
And luxury.
Because I am
a Goddess.
An Empress.
A High Priestess.

No man is the sun
that I orbit around.
I am the sun.
And the moon.
I am the entire universe,
made manifest.

I will gladly sit on the
throne by my damn self.
I am the divine feminine.
And the divine masculine.
I need nor want
for no man.
Only to be in tune with
My highest self.
Better in tune with the infinite.

I welcome my dream home!
And celebrate my transition
to a healthier lifestyle, healthier
relationships— with boundaries
with peace, love,
and serenity.

I welcome abundance.
And happiness.
I radiate joy, peace, and love.

A Message to My 25 Year Old Self

1. Get your own space.

2. You will need a sacred, quiet, clean place to make love and magic. Always have your own space even when you think you've found the man of your dreams and y'all have the ideal living situation—you need your own.

3. Don't ever get in a relationship that you an afford to leave. Always have your own. Men will always put their interests before your needs.

4. If you rely on a man to eat—He will starve you until you realize you haven't eaten in months, been full or fed.

5. It is abusive to expect or rely on anyone else to provide for you what you cannot provide for yourself.

6. To settle is to lose Self.

7. Rise; Don't fall in love.

Can I turn this poisonous relationship into a loving, fulfilling partner-
ship:
X of Wands

Is Jackson the love of my life, or did I settle:
Knight of Cups

I look at him these days and I'm so disgusted that I barely recognize him.
And I mean, he can't stand me. It's bad energy every time.
He comes home from work,
He says it's me,
I know it's him.
He said I need to be his peace when
he comes home from work,
but everyday he
brings a hurricane
home and I don't
even have an umbrella.

If being with a Black man
requires all this laying down and dying,
I'm good.
I'd much rather
Love
Myself.

I am the Empress.
Divine.
Abundance.
Fertile harvest.
Pure.

The *X of Wands* reveals that it will
Take much work to
turn our relationship healthy and whole.
Pick up the pieces.
But be careful because
You may be the only one
struggling to do so,

And blindly.

You don't need a
Knight in shining armor
To save you,
You Beautiful Queen.

If the knight isn't doing his job—replace him.
Simple.

He's made great effort to win you, but
if that isn't good enough,

Dismiss him.

January 26, 2020

I am confident. I am grateful.
I will own my own dream home in 2020.
I am healthy and happy.
I am cancer-free.
I am prosperous.
I've already won.

I've suffered great loss, heartbreak,
Pain, dis-ease. But I am whole.
I am unbroken. I am speaking
And living my truth.

I am open and receiving
everything that I've always
dreamed of!
There is no other way!
Let it be. Let it be.

I will be a homeowner!
I will be wealthy!
I am. I am. I am deserving.
I've already won.

I've pulled the knives out
Of my back and will be
Rewarded for my victory.
There is no other way.

Thank you!

January 26, 2020

So Kobe Bryant died today.
Him and his daughter in a
Tragic helicopter crash.
How wild is this game.

8-24-12-5-9

We are continuously grieving
It's almost like
these big figures are
created and
their deaths hit us
in such a capacity
that it is felt within our
Melanin.
Our skin as
Black people
In America.

We lose our heroes—daily.

I think about Jasmine all day, all the time.
And Kristina, still.
I even just tried to write her name
Like I remember
Her handwriting still.
And Jasmine's voice.
And laugh.
All in my head.

Coping Mechanisms for Grieving
the Death of a Friend:

- Sit in silence with a memory of them to honor them and acknowledge your feelings of loss and friendship.
- Breathe. Release. Any tension. Cry. Write. Run. Create. Don't sit with it.
- Honor their memory. Take up an activity they liked.
- Celebrate your friendship. Tell others about them.
- Repeat as needed.

My childhood self grieves for

Kristina
Mitchell
Aaliyah
Lisa Left Eye Lopes
Biggie
Tupac
Grandma

My young adult self grieves for

Jasmine, my lovely roomie who died of stomach cancer
Deidre, my mentor who died postpartum
Akshak, the woman who introduced me to Buddhism
James Baldwin, stomach cancer
Mike Brown
Trayvon Martin
Tamir Rice
Kendrick Johnson

I grieve now for Toni Morrison.

Life is cyclical.
At each phase or transition
We experience tragic loss

I pray it inspires us to
Continue the wheel of fortune.
And give it our best at all times.
Be the best you. Now

Literally, go.
Bye!

Question: Why did Princess Jasmine stay with Aladdin after he lied about who he was?

Did she settle?

How did she deal with the betrayal? Did she stay? Have his babies? Marry him? FORGIVE him?

Does society teach men to lie about who they are to get with women who are out of their league?

Do they spend the rest of their lives living as this fake person?

Like how women are taught to aspire to date/ marry w e a l t h y (powerful) men? (like Princess Jasmine) — **Love is *not* enough.** I used to think it was too. They tell us it is so we accept the bare minimum as soon as we hear—I love you.

Can *"i love you"* also be a spell because what is your love if you don't respect me?

Your *"i love you"* becomes a slap in the face, a mockery to the holy feminine.

January 30, 2020

I overcame the death of my best friend and roomie.
I overcame domestic violence.
I overcame poverty.
I overcame police violence.
I overcame community violence.
I overcame scarcity.
I overcame willful ignorance.
I radiate peace.
I radiate love.
I choose love instead of heartbreak.
I dream of warmth and sunlight.
I dream of a happy, healthy, village.
I dream, I dream
I dream bigger.
I welcome bigger abundance
In the form of a house.
My dream home.
Money and a car.
I will receive all of this
In 2020.

I will not be moved or shaken.
Cancer cannot stop me from my goals.
I am recovered.
I am healed.
We are healed.

FAITH
I will reach Africa.
I will cultivate cannabis.
I will heal people.
I will teach babies and moms.
I will get everything
I've dreamed of.

My Dream Home 2020

Master Suite
1-2 Guest rooms
Boys room and playroom
Beautiful backyard

Warm, sunny, open, clean modern home.

Million-dollar interior design!
Lavish, beautiful peaceful paradise
Land/Garden /Outdoor patio

A beautiful oasis to praise and thank my ancestors for guiding me.

With the sweetness of honey
on my fingertips— I am
Reminded of Oshun.

My whole life I've been giving, giving, giving.
As Black women are taught to always be in service to others.

Now is the decade I start receiving, receiving, receiving.
—love
—money
—wealth and property
—respect

To be able to receive openly
I must tune into the
Divine Feminine:

I acknowledge my worth
And the luxury and praise that I deserve and am due!
Place me upon MY throne.
Or I will have no more of this
Like Oshun.

Mind
Childbirth Education
Cannabis

Body
Pole fitness
Yoga
Herbs
Nutrition

Spirit
Sacred retreats/ womb gatherings
Reiki
Crystals
Sound healing

2.2.2020

Today is a magical day.

I am open to receiving .
The universe is teaching me
to forgive. We are human.
We have to have mercy
and understanding.
Compassion is the essence of the human spirit.

I have to forgive Jackson
And stop punishing him continuously
For hurting me and failing to
Meet the abusive standards I set for him.
It is abusive to expect—
or solely depend on a person.
I did that to him because
I was taught to,
And he allowed it because
He was taught to.

We have to do the same unlearning here.
We have to be forgiving and merciful
With each other.
So here.
I haven't been sleeping with Jackson.
I'm setting boundaries.
We have to be intimate in the mind before the physical.
We have to start all the way over.

Sometimes I question what love is,
But I know
it's unconditional.
I don't usually recognize it but it's ever present.
All encompassing.
I wanted the perfect love story
And I didn't get it.

But how or why could I expect perfection
in such an imperfect world.
Happiness exists within me.
As long as I have me
I have love and happiness

So the question this whole time
of whether to stay or leave Jackson
has not really been a question of necessarily being here
or being together physically,
or sharing the same space but
whether I choose me, first.

And I do,
I do, I do.

Wedding Vows to Myself

I promise, everyday to choose you first.
I promise to support and love you entirely,
mind, body, and spirit.
I promise to only feed you truth.
I promise to stay committed to growth
and guidance from the ancestors, the Creator, and the universe.
I promise to be light and speak truth to power.
I promise to nourish you with fresh water, fresh organic produce,
herbs and quality cannabis.
I promise to water you and breathe with you.
I promise to hold my ground in defending and protecting you.
I promise to provide and protect you.
I promise to serve you.
I will love you forever and will
birth a wondrous, prosperous,
and wealthy life for you.

You are the empress, your highness.
You are the Queen, many moons over.
You are the divine Ma'at.
The sacred balance of the universe
for which all things begin and end.

I honor you, Black Wombman.
To thee, I wed forever and ever.

Asé.

My words will be more powerful than Malcolm X
More truthful than James Baldwin
More eloquent than Maya
More beautiful than Toni
Like Water for Chocolate City

"Let the experience teach you
And be real—

And there will be warfare involved."
- Lauryn Hill Unplugged : Interlude 5

I've been at war since I first embarked on this journey—
that day I decided, sitting there in Barnes and Noble.

I'm here now on 2.2.20.
I've won.
We made it out whole.
With new ways of relating to one another.
This is me.

"Every tub has to stand on its own bottom."

So here I stand, strong, more resilient,
more powerful and fearless,
standing in my truth.
Sharing my story, healing from the inside out.

We don't have to be
on the same page, or even in the
same book.

We can be in different books, on different shelves,
in different rooms…what matters, truly,
is that we come together in the same house,
to share the innermost truth
that our own books contain.

This is my book.

(I get out of all your boxes)

So often we enter relationships
expecting the other person to help
us carry, sort, and fix all of our shit.
Literally two people,
dumping piles of shit,
years of baggage onto each other.
Between one another.

Instead,
have the will to sort through
your own shit, fixing what you
can, getting help and support when
you need—not depending on the
other person to do that with you or for you.
They can sort their shit
next to you, offering what
wisdom they've gained.
Nor do you take on the responsibility
of fixing them, sorting them, organizing them.

They do not belong to you.

You belong to you alone.
When two people come together
in the same house, sorting through themselves,
supporting one another,
climbing,
Leaving no one behind.

Revolutionary love.

Things I've Learned While Smoking Weed:
A Message to My 25 year old Self

To the girl in my twenties
To the girl in my teens
To my younger Self

1. Don't forget who you are and where you stand in the struggle.
2. Some men will spend the rest of their lives kissing your feet, because that all they deserve.
3. Lauryn Hill, Unplugged is soul food. India. Arie, Voyage to India is soul food for the Black Girl Soul. Like Water for Chocolate City.
4. Find a dependable man (partner) who loves you. Let him love you, but don't depend on him.
5. Compassion is the essence of the human spirit. We have to be merciful with one another. That's empathy and understanding and love.
6. Love is not all you need.
7. You need respect
8. You need loyalty
9. You need truth
10. You need water, cannabis, and quality food.
11. You need luxurious living accommodations, as a bare minimum
12. Don't settle for less than you deserve. (see above, love is not all you need)
13. Breathe.
14. Love
15. Release
16. Never stop moving. Water that stops flowing freely becomes stale.
17. Never let people suck you dry or dry you out. The Divine Feminine is always wet. And overflowing in abundance.
18. Choose you, first. Marry yourself first. Say you do to your damn self. (I do!)
19. Make sure you are married to your dreams and the life you have created for yourself instead of waiting for someone to help create a life with you.
20. Only you can journey on your path— everyone else is around you as a bonus. Be grateful for real friends and the ones who love you.

21. Carry your ancestors with you everywhere.
22. Remember Kristina, when you talk to teen girls about their bodies, sex, boys, and self-esteem.
23. Remember Jasmine, when you talk to women and girls about nutrition, natural holistic remedies and cannabis.
24. Remember Mama Deirdre, when you support women and birthing families have healthy, happy families
25. Remember who you are and all the Happy Brown Babies that will be born in joy and peace because of you. All life began with you.
26. Be the driver on the road to pursuing your dream— you drive.
27. Don't settle for or get complacent in the passenger seat

Congratulations!

What will I gain in 2020?

All the joy in the world
And a big, beautiful, luxurious dream house.

#LoveisNOTallyouneed
#LoveBigger #DreamBigger

When I get
my dream house
I will spend the
REST of my life helping Black people get their dream home!

Thank you!

I am a winner!
I won!

2.5.2020

I pulled *The Devil* card the other day and was trying to figure out what bad habit and addictions I may have been slipping back into. Took me a couple days:

Meat: I tend to eat more flesh when I'm stressed the fuck out especially when Jackson and I get into it or things aren't feeling right or when I'm on my period. So I was heavily consuming meat over the last few days. I release that energy. It made me completely fatigued and tired.

I need fresh fruit and vegetables.
Smoothies and herbs.
I want nothing else.

How can I manifest a healthier relationship to food?

I need this in order to live.
So I accept nothing less. I just won't eat.

I release being too forgiving!
As I said, some people will spend the rest of their life kissing your feet because that's all they deserve.

I'm releasing Jackson and his mom
and the dysfunction I found myself in,
I release it.

This will continue if I forgive Jackson and his family.
They will continue to collectively disrespect me.
That's how domestic violence works.
It masquerades around with no boundaries and
constantly spews out sarcastic remarks and shameful
comments disguised as advice.

When you grow up in such dysfunction,
you don't readily notice what's going on.

It just feels normal, comfortable.
I know that if I want to break the curse,
I have to stay far away from what feels
normal and comfortable.

So I have to keep it moving.

I release myself to the universe
to supply my needs and deepest desires—
whether spoke or unspoken.

I've decided this current life no longer serves me.
I accept better.
I command better.

I command respect.
I command compassion.
I command unconditional love.
I command luxury and wealth.
I command peace.
I command holistic healing.

Lessons I had to learn the hard way—

so you won't have to:

1. Don't look for money in all the wrong places

This is a lesson that I carry with me, as part of my journey to woman-hood. Most women experience this but don't teach other women how *not* to do what they did—so I hope this helps some twenty to twenty-five year old who is going through that naive period in a girl's journey where we are often tricked by men (or women who work for them) into doing something that we wouldn't normally do because we need money. This is also a lesson in making sure you have your own money. This is not an easy experience or lesson and is not one that will be easy to tell. I've told no one this. But I release it here, so that you may be healed.

I was sitting on the subway platform one evening after I had just quit my job. I was coming home from the grocery store with a ton of groceries—my last shopping trip, the last of my savings. I was looking for a job—desperately. Rent was past due. Maybe it was obvious. So a Latino man comes up to me and tells me he just left work, and that he gives massages at a parlor. He makes small talk and tells me they are hiring. I was like yes. It must be a sign from the universe. A job, right on time.

So he tells me to call him in the morning and we'll talk more. I call him in the morning and he's like, "yeah meet me at this Metro station, we can do a training, and I'll give your information to my boss and let her know I trained you."

To me it sounded like a great opportunity to help people. Massage ther-apy is awesome. So I agreed.

Got to the train station, and I called him. He's on the phone telling me directions to where he is, I walk down the block, up the street, over this way and that way. He's having me call him every time I make it to each new destination. I end up walking maybe ten minutes to a house where I see the guy. I'm like, okay…why didn't he just give me the address, instead of having me call him? He looked harmless, and was nice to me.

So he leads me in a small basement apartment where an elderly Latina woman is cooking. She can't speak English. It's his mom.
I say, "Hola."
She's sweet, and continues cooking.

On the other side of the kitchen is a sheet dividing the room, behind the sheet is a bed.
He explains it's where he sleeps.
He instructs me to massage him to let him see what I can do, if I can do the job.
I do not do a good job.
He tries to get me to massage his penis.
This grown ass man, living in his moms kitchen behind a sheet, with Jergen's lotion.
His penis is the size of my thumb.
I've never seen one so small.
He can tell by the look on my face.

"What? You've only been with Black dudes?" he asks, then tells me I'm not doing it right, so he shows me. He massages me with lotion.
Massaged my whole body and then tried to give me head!
It was not working! NOT working!
He was embarrassed.
I grabbed my things.
He apologized.
He said he was in a bad place and was trying to get his wife and kids back.

I left out that place so quick.

Women and girls get trafficked without even realizing it. Men don't have to physically move us, we do it ourselves. There are many lessons here.

Be weary of men who offer something that seems to good to be true— it is.

Run— from men with little penises.

Don't look for money where you ain't never found none before.

I realized my naivety.
And released any shame and guilt I had from this experience.
It was the first time I douched in a tub of hot water.

I'm thankful that he didn't violate me even more by raping me or demanding head.

This happened when I was 24.
I know worst things that have happened to girls at this age who find themselves in situations with little money and resources.

2. Don't look for love in all the wrong places.
(i.e. don't ignore the red flags)

It's so easy, almost instinctual to look for love in familial places. But when familiar places are toxic, abusive, and unhealthy it may be more beneficial to look for love in unfamiliar, new places. Outside of our comfort zones. And even when we get there, don't ignore the red flags, just because the are "new" red flags!

In fact, I don't look for love at all.

Because you will attract love.
It's when you go look for it is when you end up finding a bunch of bullshit, disguised as this idea of love that we have in our heads (and that's probably not the most healthy perception of love.)

The type of love that I was searching for, of course, I had within myself. The thing is, attracting (not finding) someone who loves themselves as much as you love yourself and who can love you just as you love yourself—if not, more.

You have to show people how to love you by loving yourself. A man will only treaty how he sees you treat yourself.

A man will never take you to eat at McDonald's if he's never seen you eat/ feed your spirit that type of food. (No shade)

366

I do believe that I was looking for love in all the wrong places, not when I first met Jackson, but when I moved back to DC and moved in with him. I was definitely searching. I was looking. I was wrong.
And I take full credit for jumping in the water and not knowing how to swim.

I'm glad I didn't drown. I could have.
I coasted for a long time, floating—half way there.
I decided to keep swimming and learn to recognize love with new eyes, in new languages.

Don't ignore the red flags (even in yourself.)
I used to ask for signs, see a fed flag and quickly put it in my pocket like I never saw it in the first place, until one day there was no more room in my pocket for anymore red flags.
There were so many red flags it was too heavy to carry.
It became my burden.
I became less than myself trying to ignore all these red flags and still be whole and loving and peaceful. It's impossible
It welcomes,
It breeds,
Illness.
A disconnect with the mind-body-spirit.

Red flags are a warning for a reason, sis.
Don't ignore them.

3. Don't go out with someone you would never go out with

This goes right in line with not ignoring the red flags. When you set your standards for the men you date— never lower them or make exceptions.
—I said I would never date another Scorpio.
—I said I would never date another Alpha.

I ignored these standards that I set and it led to red flag, after red flag. But I *knew* better.

This is a lesson I've learned many times over in many different relationships with men and women. This is the lesson that teaches the importance of setting boundaries and standards in friendships and relationships. I learned this lesson the hard way when I was raped by a guy who one of my line sisters considered to be her best friend.

I said I would never go out with him.

Jerrod knew I'd never give him the time of day. He took advantage of me one drunk night in college but he raped me after that, one summer in Chicago in 2015. I think to this day, I only told a few people but it was a big lesson. I said I would never go out with him, then he kept hanging around my sister. I decided to give him the benefit of the doubt. We went to an art show in Bronzeville with another couple then to a comedy show. A real clown the whole night. I had wine, like my usual. Not enough to forget or be off my ass.

I don't remember getting in a cab and going to his place.
But I remember being there.
I remember smoking one hit of something then waking up to him fucking my body.

Literally.
I woke up and he was having sex with me.
I remember in that moment looking around the room in such shock and confusion.
His room was trashed and disgusting.
I fell back out.
Then woke up to him saying,
"I'm going to work—bye Melanie."
He leaves— I hear the front door close. I rush to put on my clothes and run out the door.
Didn't know where I was walking for ten minutes.

Then I walked into Hyde Park Produce and bought more groceries than I could carry home. Then I carried them all the way back to where I was staying with my sister and her roommates. I took a bath in their bathtub and cried myself to sleep on the room floor.

"Did you at least use a condom?" I texted him.
He replied, "of course not, why would I do that?"

He bragged about how wet I was, how I came so many times. I was embarrassed that my body confused him into forgetting that he was raping me. He put something in my drink. Probably the last glass of wine he got up to get me at the comedy show instead of ordering with the waiter at our table—he got up and came back with another glass. I drank it and that's all I remember until the scene in the cab, the scene in his living room, them waking up to him fucking me.

I take ownership in that I should have never gone out with him. I knew the type of man that he was. That he raped Kalaya in college. I went because I wanted to go on a date. I lowered my standard and I learned a very valuable lesson that I hope you won't have to learn the hard way.

That lesson was also one teaching me to also break ties with the line sister that considered him to be her best friend. As this stood, she never held him accountable for the fuck shit he did to many women. I never told her.

Because she is one of those women—
it doesn't matter how many women hate him.
He ended up getting some girl pregnant not long after that happened to me and I had idea about how that may have happened. I'm just thankful it wasn't me.

My sister and I went to get tested.
Three days after it happened.

I told a few close friends.
I'm telling you so you'll learn to never
go out with anyone
you'd never go out with.

And no,
it's never too late to tell.

Release it.
#metoo

2.10.20

I want so badly to just go.
Surrounded by warmth
It's too cold here.
It was too cold in Baltimore.
And in Chicago.

I yearn for vitamin D!
I know that it is coming.
Everything that I need and want,
spoken and unspoken
will come to be.
In due time.
For my maximum benefit.
Until then, I will continue to practice gratitude.

I'm grateful for the women that have come
before me, knowing them helps to know who I am,
where I belong
and why.

I want to know so bad.
I thought the emptiness I felt was from not having my own family,
when it was actually not knowing my family's roots.
Our maternal lineage.

Reading these slave narratives, thinking about what I learned on line
really makes sense. I have to learn my mom's lineage.
My mission in life is to become a midwife. Help birth happy, beautiful,
healthy babies into the world. Free babies.

I want to birth babies into a world I can be proud of.
There is so much darkness. If I could be one of light then I could truly
understand my purpose for being here.

I want / I desire the luxury to love, teach, and nourish my boys with no worries of finances. I want a beautiful home for us to grow up in. (which sounds a lot like words I'd written in my journal as a girl)

How long have I been yearning for a safe, clean, loving, beautiful home? —29 years (almost 30!)

My life is ending as I know it.

The universe is bringing a new way of life. I'm rejecting all things that I once considered love, all that I once considered normal. Because I deserve better than that. I deserve to love a *healed* man. A mature man. A loving man. A king. I've been waiting too long. Waiting—for some man to save me? I am my own hero.

I want to provide for my family.
I want to live a healthy lifestyle.
I want to be surrounded by lush bountiful nature,
Where my boys can run and be fat.

I'll never have too much pride to bring my ass home to my mom.
I'm just so ready to move forward.
I deserve trips to Jamaica and whole blogs dedicated to loving me.
I deserve flowers and plants every week.
I deserve it all without asking.
The universe will match my energy
and send me all that I attract in love and peace.
And remove all that DOES NOT serve me!

I release all that I've been hanging on to
just because I didn't want to be alone.
My little ones deserve better and so do I.

February 14

Nevermind it's Valentine's Day.

A few days ago I watched a Netflix documentary,
 "Who Killed Malcolm X?"

I was hesitant to watch it at first because I figured it'd be triggering and
it was. It's like a question I'd had all my life was finally answered and in
great detail—
It's been on my mind since I watched it
I'm more determined than ever to leave this country,
to return home to Africa to live our greatest lives!

I will be successful in midwifery.
I will be successful in real estate.
I will be successful in cannabis.
I will be successful in family services.
I will be a successful educator.

I am wealthy.
I am abundant.
I am melanin.

Healing

Mind:

Therapist
Books
Journal

Body:

Fresh fruit/ veggies
Juicer / Blender / Food Processor
Herbs: Sea Moss, Bladderwrack, Sarsaparilla
Detox
Cannabis regime
Yoga
Pole fitness
Weights

Spirit

Reiki
Sound Bowls
Crystals

SLEEP
I need sleep.

What happens when you take a giraffe
out of its natural habitat (in Africa)
And bring him to a zoo in North America?

How do they adapt?
How do they change?

What would happen
Upon returning to
Africa?

Over time, giraffes born in captivity probably
think it's their natural habitat.

How long have they wanted to go home?

What about their family (tribe) in Africa?

Make communities in Africa for returning giraffes.

2.15.20

There is magic in my blood.
The ashes of my ancestors is in my bones.

I will manifest my dream home on an island, catching, and educating babies traveling to and from Africa, saving giraffes, writing, and telling the stories of the African people who were kidnapped from the shores of our Motherland and forced into slavery, chattel slavery, bought and sold as commodity, for hundred of years building corporations in every industry we know today, all over the world.

A people who had their language, history, and religion wiped away. A people who endured genocide through psychological, medical warfare and domestic terrorism, abuse and racism.

A people who's leaders continue to be assassinated, manipulated, and infiltrated. I will tell everyone how they colluded to kill our Black Messiah— The Honorable Malik El-Hajj Shabazz. I will tell them of James Baldwin, of the Black Panther Party, Toni Morrison, of Maya Angelou, of Assata, of political prisoners, of The People! The MOVE Organization.

As far as America to Africa everyone will know OUR TRUE STORY and Melanin & Books.

I will support women and babies in Africa.

I will be a renowned, published author and educator.

I will grow cannabis and teach Black people all over the world about how to heal with cannabis.

I will cure my own illnesses.

I will build an design homes for Black people all over the world, especially women and children.

I will be healthy, wealthy, happy, joyful, and wise.

I will enjoy peace and sunshine.

I will enjoy my home as paradise and praise the Goddess for love and abundance.

Everyone will know the truth with my words and their lives will be enriched forever through my books and the story of my life.

I will keep going until I reach the shores of Africa, then and only then

I will dance and celebrate my journey.

2.22.2020

My *Holistic Cannabis Consumption: Pregnancy, Childbirth, & Postpartum online course* is launching in 3 days!

I am so proud of myself!
Turning poison into medicine and leaving no one behind.

Ode to my ancestors.
That's alchemy.
Turning the poison into
Fuel to drive our mission
Forward.

I applied for a small business grant and I am confident that I will win. I am thankful for the partnerships and donations that I've received and I will continue to share my story and my mission to reverse karma and enjoy life in freedom. True freedom—from the inside, out.

10 people paid for my class!
More are coming!

2.23.20

I am healed.
Recovery is beautiful.

Did you know the braiding hair Kanekelon is a synthetic plastic fiber that is not safe, maybe a carcinogen, and definitely shouldn't be in our heads?

Who created this knowing only Black women use this product?

In order to heal we have to look at what making us sick...

My salt water bath allowed me to release those things.

I know what I need to heal.

Healers need healers.

And love.
Of which I've been
feeling very little
from anyone other than my babies.

I welcome a stronger, better love.
A dependable, spiritual, deep love.
Rooted in truth and respect and honesty.

I want a man who loves me, deeply.
I want a king who will sit beside me on *my* throne.
Who will praise me and lift me up.
Hold me, up and down.
Who will pray over me.
Meditate and elevate
with me—our physical bodies holding
no barriers to our connection.
I want to be the earth, the sun,

and the moon.
And he project the masculine
of my feminine.
I want wealth of my own,
my own kingdom.
The crown is mine.

All that is mine
is due to me.
And I welcome it.
I want a man, a true king, who
is healthy, wealthy, and wise.
Supportive, gentle, and kind.
Passionate, but also compassionate,
Confident and courageous.
Independent, humble, strong, and skilled.
I welcome you.

I must welcome these in myself so that
they may manifest in the physical.

February 28th

My great-grandma, Grams, was born in 1904 or 1906. She lived in South Blytheville Arkansas. She gave birth to 14 children, 7 lived to adulthood. My grandma, Theretha, was number 11 overrall, but was number 5 of the 7. Grams had children die in infancy of whooping cough and pneumonia. One child drowned, tragically. She was said to have cried often for her babies. She gave birth to 14 babies and had no stretch marks. She said you had to put oil on your skin. She used vaseline, mineral oil, and cocoa butter. She was short, petite and fat and made a bomb lemon cake. She was a midwife. She gave birth to half the world, if you let her tell it. She put Royal Crown in her hair. She loved to drink and was a conspiracy theorist. She lived to be 90 years and 18 days old. Midwifery was in her blood, and in her heart. She cried up until she died about not being able to go to nursing school to be a licensed midwife to work in hospitals.

She could smell pregnancy. Grams could even tell when the baby ain't belong to the daddy.

One day, cousin Lisa and my Auntie Dennis came in the house from outside, Grams said, "You pregnant, ain't you Lisa?"
Lisa said, "I'm saved, sanctified, and filled with the Holy Ghost!"
Grams looked at her, "You filled with something, but it ain't yo husband's, huh Lisa?" Grams was talking bout the baby she was pregnant with wasn't her husband's baby! And come to find out, she was pregnant and it wasn't his baby.

Grams was raised Baptist and was considered "The Mother" of the Baptist Church she went to. Mother Francis. She lived by *The Good Book*. She knew everything it said, and would be quick to tell on the pastor for trying to get money from the congregation by saying it was written in the bible. Her father was partly, or maybe full Native American, but lived as a Black man due to the unjust treatment of Natives at the time.

"Everyone would look down on me when I was a teenager, and I got pregnant," Auntie Dennis told me about the first time she had sex and got pregnant at sixteen. Grams told her, "Get up guhh, get up! Have you ever seen somebody walk up side somebody?"

"Nah, I ain't never seen that," Auntie Dennis replied confusedly.

Grams said, " In order for somebody to walk all over you, you have to agree to lay down."

"She didn't talk to me like I was stupid, like I didn't know." Auntie said about Grams and how she supported her during pregnancy. You know how a lot of women would fix a man's plate before feeding their children, not Grams. And everybody wanted seconds of Grams' food. One day that same pastor came over at dinner and tried to tell Grams that she had to fix his plate before her grandchildren. Grams never gave anybody seconds, but you better believe she gave the children seconds and thirds that day, before the pastor ate anything. Grams ain't play.

She never let men eat before children.

She said we can't raise our kids like white folks. When you get pregnant, you have to eat real food, Southern food, our food. You were to wear a girdle after birth and stay in for 30 days, or it'll catch up with you later when you turn 43.

When Roe vs. Wade passed, Grams broke down crying.

She said it was an act of genocide and that they gone make us pay for all these abortions. Not us meaning the women getting the abortions, but the U.S. for passing a law giving women the choice to "act as God." She didn't trust medicalized abortions, she considered it to be eugenics.

Grams gave birth to four generations of nurses.

Her daughter, Aunt Bert, was a Head Surgical Nurse in California, my Auntie Brenda became an LPN and my cousin, a Nurse Practitioner. And on my dad's side, I have two aunts with PhDs in Nursing, and even more cousins who are nurses or once aspired to be one. It's in the blood.

Grams would mix up herbs; she had a concoction for everything, and they worked every time. When Aunt Bert gave birth early to her oldest daughter Tina, the doctors said she wasn't gone make it. Grams said she had to go up to the hospital to go get her baby, because the doctors didn't know what they were doing. Cousin Tina was a preemie, back when premature babies did not live.

Grams took that baby home, fed that baby, and gave that baby some of her herbs. Now imagine if Grams didn't go up there and they had just listened to the doctors. Cousin Tina went on to have two children of her own, and they have children. And the doctors tried to say she wasn't gone make it.

I pray for the privilege and honor of becoming a midwife in the honor and legacy of my Grams, Mary Francis Evans Love Robinson Collins.

I will raise my boys in another country.

The men in this country (read: Black men in this country) have been failed by their mothers. They were kept away from their fathers then were expected to be their mom's boyfriend or best friend. They were either feminized or hyper-masculinized from their trauma—made into the toxic males we see and love today.

They've been married to their moms—in emotionally abusive relationships, where they've been the protector, even the provider, picking her up after every bad break up. They've been the best friend she's never had. These little boys. Children.

They've been raped by their mother's friends, or babysitters, or cousins, women old enough to be their mother, or women their mothers sent to make a "man" out of them. These women. These mothers who allow their sons to abuse other women. These women who teach their sons to abuse women by allowing men to abuse them and expecting their child to save them. There are so many women like this who have 30+ year old sons who hate them. Either secretly enraged or have outright hate toward Black women. These are the men we sleep with at night, who we've had children with. These men who secretly hate their mothers. For keeping their fathers away, or for not being kept. For all the things.

How can they ever love us completely if they hate their moms so much?

I deserve the world.

Healing generational trauma is healing mother-son and father-daughter wounds that roots back to slavery.

We carry luggage that doesn't even belong to us.

I'm attracting a healed, whole family.
A healed, healthy, whole partner, lover with a healthy relationship with his mother and all women. I deserve more. I'm providing for and protecting myself until the Divine Masculine is worthy to receive me. I deserve divine, earth-shattering love.

I deserve to be swept off to Africa.
I deserve my palace, on my throne.
I deserve the world.

Praises be to Seshat as I continue
to teach on the sacred cannabis plant.

May you continue to move through me.

Asé

3.4.2020

I know.
I need to focus on my self-care.
It's been practically a year since the thyroid cancer diagnosis and I have yet to start my cannabis treatment (or even detox my body.) I've been so focused on building Happy Brown Baby and The Cannabis Doula, and training with various organizations. I'm tired. I have nothing to give, no energy. Even my arm is weak, tired of writing.

I need more than a vacation.
I deserve a complete change in my surroundings. If I am in a place that does not support me—I release it.

This is bullshit.
I've worked so fucking hard to be where I am and I am still lacking the wealth necessary to heal my body and fully live in my purpose. I'm fucking tired of fighting and struggling to live.
Struggling to eat, to medicate.
Struggling to be! I'm fucking done.

This week (it's only Wednesday) I've been pushed to the edge.
I don't know who to trust.
Me and Jackson.
I don't know what the fuck this is.
We argue everyday.
He can't see how his dysfunctional relationship with his mom affects our relationship. This really sucks. I never wanted to raise boys who see and hear their dad disrespect me daily.
I literally had to get out of the car, in the freezing cold, at night because he wouldn't stop yelling at me.
I walked for probably an hour with no phone, to the mall and had dinner, because I hadn't eaten all day. I enjoyed my wine, then walked back toward the house.
It was 9:30pm.
I got out the car at 6:30pm.

As I was walking, they pulled up behind me.
It was so cold.

But this isn't the first time I got out of the car because Jackson was tripping. The day I spoke at the Women Grow Leadership Summit, my phone died. I came out 30mins after I said for him to pick me up. I called him from someone's phone. He cursed me out. Got in the car, he curses me out from DC to Silver Spring. By the time we got near the house, I couldn't take it so I got out the car and started walking. He then stops, gets out the car, and proceeds to yell and tell me to get the boys. Can you imagine?
So, I get the stroller and the boys and he pulls the fuck off.

We roam the neighborhood, for hours.

I was preparing to sleep in a park bench with two babies. My phone was dead and I had no money.
He said he'd never do it again.
But, it happened again.
The only reason he didn't tell me to get the boys this time was because it was 30 degrees outside.

Why am I here?

I don't eat shit.
My skin is breaking out.
I'm not happy,
I moved my mattress back into my meditation room.

He leaves no money, or food for the boys.
How does he not leave money, ever?
He's been "broke" the moment he asked me to be in a relationship with him.
All of a sudden he can't afford anything.
I just want to know where the money goes.
The refrigerator is always empty. I have to do the most bitch
Just to get money to go to Trader Joes.
This can't be it.

How many generations of my family have been struggling for food, and with domestic violence?

Kill it, please.
Release me from this karma.
Or kill me.
I cannot exist as this person. In this life. Any more.
I fucking hate it here.

I'm trying to decide if I should postpone my early childhood education classes.

Should I leave?

He's so mean,
it's killing me.

Full Moon | 3.9.2020

I am open and receiving all the needs and desires of my heart.

I washed away poverty, scarcity, and lack.

I welcome riches and wealth in the form of money, property, and resources.

I have and welcome an abundance of healthy, organic food—fruit, vegetables, fresh water, and land to reap harvest after harvest for generations.

I accept full responsibility for my wealth and will positivity shift the culture. I will change lives and heal with my words, my work, and my love.

For my Happy Brown Babies.

3.14.20

I feel like my heart has been cut out
of my chest and thrown in the garbage.

I hate Jackson so much.
I hate his mom even more.
And I am happy to finally release the burden of these emotions.
I was looking for love in all the wrong places—but I refuse to stay in this
wrong, loveless place.

I am worthy of love and kindness.
I am worthy of respect.
Someone's love and respect for you should not depend on what you can
do for them or because of your relationship to someone else.

I could kill him.
I could kill myself.
I could leave forever and never look back.
All things I've considered.
Our relationship is over.
Our family is done.

It was over before it started and it's hard for me not to believe he planned
to ruin my life the moment he saw me.

3.15.20

I have decisions to make.
And a flight to LA on April 1st.

It's a new chapter.
I'm determined.
Anything I want I can have and I will.

A big home in a beautiful neighborhood in a city that I adore surrounded by people who love and support me.

That's all I've been in search for this whole time.
I'm determined. I have two months to do what I love and make money.

I need a solid foundation for the boys and I cannot do that under Jackson and his mom. We need our own. Jackson needs to do whatever it is he needs to do, away from me for however long, and maybe I'll be able to heal and forgive.
And love,
And trust
again, one day.

Until then—I'm making love to myself.

I'm going to Cali!

3.18.20

I refuse to be reduced by fear.
I will conquer.
My dream home is coming.
The life I deserve to live is weeks away.
I refuse to be controlled by fear
Of any virus.
Of any man.
Of any thing.

I have the money I need and the land and resources to protect and provide for my family.

We are not here to suffer.
I radiate joy, peace, and understanding.
I am light.
I am truth.
I am invincible.
I am God.

Everything I need and want is mine.
I have money, land, and my dream home.
I am abundant and well.

Everything that no longer serves me is dead.
I accept abundance in every form.

I will share my story and change the lives
Of girls and women everywhere.

I am a powerful speaker.

I am a brilliant writer.
My work will be compared to Toni Morrison, Maya Angelou,
and Nikki Giovanni. Everyone will know me.

3.26.2020

I affirm and center my whole health and wellness.
I am grateful for the healing and the herbs that will aid my journey.
I am grateful for the Creator, for Allah.
For restoring me.
And for gifting me with purpose.
Purpose to heal and love through
Light and truth,
I am the greatest version of myself.
I am melanin.
I am God.
I am the transparent enlightenment
of my own rebirth.
I am like water for chocolate city.

My cannabis business and brand will be an internationally acclaimed business. I will make millions of dollars in my CBD products, classes, and consultations. I will have my own CBD shop with books centering women and families holistic health.

The Diaspora.

I am grateful and humbled by my ancestors. We've been quarantined and practicing social distancing and being told to stay in our homes. Schools are closed. No sporting events or amusement parks. No cruise ships. Only essential businesses are operating and medical and essential persons are sill going to work. No library. Grocery stores are lacking most essentials because of people panic shopping. Everything is a limited commodity. COVID-19 is killing people, from China, to Europe, and now they are telling us to prepare. Like the wind is all of a sudden going to blow and become toxic and we'll just start dropping like flies. While that sounds like an unlikely occasion it may just happen. Not only is this virus a strategy of war, this may very well be a plan to help Trump win the next election. The US has a patent on the virus and Europe has a patent on the vaccine. Until I can amass enough wealth to escape this country, we will all be vulnerable, our health put at risk for the control and power of a few. People are very much losing their lives.

I speak truth over my family and friends that we are not disillusioned by fear. I speak protection and comfort. I pray for all birthing people during this time and pray that babies are guided and welcomed into this world with joy.

If the whole world has to be
made new,
washed clean
in order for wealth
to be redistributed
for power to be exposed
for humanity to be
broken
open,
I am here for it.

I am here for the radical change
That will shift my whole existence,
For generations.
I welcome the wealth of my
Ancestor's hard work.

Radical | Revolutionary | Shifting

Do you feel it?

The world is mine.

April 2nd

Our flight would have landed in California.
Yesterday.
For two months.
But it was canceled much like all other flights. Stay-at-home orders have been mandated, other countries are sending in medical supplies, states are bracing for the worst; turning some places into temporary hospitals. People are dying. People are losing their jobs. Schools are closing for the year. The whole world has shifted. People are realizing the gaps in medical care and quality of life here in the U.S.

Cannabis will be the new medicine.
They will recognize how cannabis inhalation is especially useful in respiratory infections...
Until then...

I know the universe has something bigger in store and will deliver my dream home and my soul mate. Even though I'm not physically able to separate, I must still emotionally and mentally break through this without having all my resources drained.

I pray for my strength.
I pray for my health and wellness.
I pray for a higher energy.
I pray for true love.
I pray for peace.
I pray for compassion.

I pray for someone who will never turn their back to me when we sleep together.

I pray for someone who doesn't sigh or roll their eyes when I speak.

I pray for someone who is kind and gentle and peaceful.

I pray for someone who loves me, for me, not for what I can do for them.

I can't remember the last time Jackson and I had sex, but I'm pretty sure it was the time I swallowed his cum and it actually tasted like a toxic shot of alcohol. Literally, that's the gag. And it dawned on me why my vagina was always fucked up after we had sex or he gave me head. Toxic af. Last night Jackson made it clear that this month makes six months, which could be true but I haven't been keeping track nor am I trying to get "accidentally" pregnant so I don't care. I've definitely been considering getting a vibrator just to prevent myself from lowering my standards. I'm sticking to it.

I have more respect and love for my womb than to destroy my pH! I cannot stand the burning/ itching. I am a queen. My yoni is sacred. I will keep her sacred until my soulmate finds me.

My heart is hurt but such is the ebb and flow of life.

If I stay, I become complacent,
And settle for much less than I will ever desire.
My plans to rebuild have been canceled.
I know the universe has better.
I am receiving.
I am abundant.

May 12, 2020

Jackson had a mouth full of blood this morning and that's exactly what the fuck he gets for not calling my mom and wishing her a happy Mother's Day, after having the fucking audacity to get mad at me for not going over his mom's house— like I have no fucking choice in how I celebrate my Mother's Day.

As if I needed another fucking sign. He's still choosing to please his mother instead of protecting me and our relationship. He chooses her every time and we get into it, every time. When will we learn.

I would never expect him to choose me over his mother—but a real man doesn't have to. A real woman would never raise her son to put herself in competition with his partner. This is why broken women cannot raise healthy men or healthy children, period.

So yes, Jackson ended up with a mouth full of blood because he doesn't listen.

He doesn't honor or respect women.
He's a narcissist, arrogant,
Scorpio who had the audacity—
The nerve—to forget to wish my mom
A happy, beautiful, blissful Mother's Day—

May you never forget this day.

A balloon, a glass vase of red roses,
A necklace, a purse
Is what he got me for Mother's Day.
First, I thought something was off with the balloon
then the roses in a glass vase.
"She wasn't impressed."
So he left, and came back with a necklace and a purse.
Better.
Maybe he doesn't think I'm a good mom.

Clearly.
He didn't wish my mom a happy Mother's Day,
But he can call her and tell her
He's only with me for the boys.

So yes, he woke up this morning and started eating me out.
He was having a nice time, doing a good job, and came up with a mouth
full of my period blood.
As if sweet Oshun herself plotted revenge on my behalf.
But this feels much better.
This could be the last time we have sex and he will never ever forget me
or forget to respect me—the wombman who birthed to him two Black
children,
and the women,
the women
who birthed me.

Had the stay at home order and COVID-19 hadn't happened, I'd be in
LA with the boys. Probably trying to build a life without Jackson and
trying to move out to Cali for good. I thought this was the universe' way
of revealing that we needed to try harder, work it out for the boys but
more so it has shown me how unhealthy and toxic our living situations
have been to the point where one of us has to be gone for at least 9 hours
in the day or longer to make our lives work.

Relationship take work. So does a relationship with one's Self.
And as far as I'm concerned, being in a loving relationship
with myself is far more important than being in a relationship just to im-
press Jackson's mom or to help him live up to whatever fantasy she has
for him. And he will very much spend the rest of his life dating his mom
and trying to make her happy.
Not I.

I gave up a long time ago
living for my parents
and this image and idea that they have for me.
I almost applied to nursing school.
And it's not even that I don't
want to be a midwife,
It's just that I do!

Learning the ways and traditions
of the women and healers
before me will not be found
within the halls of white
hospitals and the classrooms of
racist institutions.

The information will appear
when I am ready to receive it.
Perhaps when my babies are older and over-loved by their own mother
will the ancestors grant me permission to mother others into this realm.

I'm still healing and have a lot of mothering to do myself,
I am journeying into sound healing And training as a yoni steam practi-
tioner. I want to open my home studio where I offer holistic doula
services, cannabis caregiver services, education, and events.
With a bomb ass library. For the Diaspora.
Our culture.
Our cannabis.
Our traditions.

I will travel the world telling stories of how
Lives have changed with a single plant.
Our countries.
Tribes
of people
in bondage. In fields.
Sowing the land
For a country and a dream that they
and their descendants—us,
would probably never see.

Enslaved African people, our ancestors,
were bought and traded with hemp.
They were master cultivators and experimented
in using all part of the cannabis plant.
Pipe smoking, originating in Africa, survived
the slave trade and manifests today,
in this country and in South America.

Cannabis is a culture of the diaspora and because people are forgetting and white people are colonizing the industry, I've been left no choice but to tell the story of how the capitalization/colonizations of hemp, the war on drugs and the prohibition of cannabis—including the buying, selling, and enslavement of my ancestors for it—led to not only the domestic violence and chronic illnesses in our communities, it has also led to our perceived lower-caste status, violence ridden, over-policed neighborhoods, poor schools… and high prison populations.

Even as medical cannabis programs are popping up in states and predominately white states are legalizing, Black people remain those who are still criminalized, arrested, and jailed for cannabis possession and related charges. Even as a medical cannabis patient—I still can't afford my medication—it was not set up for us.

All of that to say this:

No one (meaning no Black person) has ever saved their own life by following the rules (written for and by white supremacist.)

I will cultivate cannabis to heal my body and my community.

My Experience at DC Growers - Junior Gardener

Apr 3, 2020, 12:33 AM

Hi Mr. Vincent,

I hope this message finds you well. I'm writing this to share some feedback with you about my experience working at DC Growers that I believe will be of value to your company and possibly other businesses in the cannabis industry. I worked at DC Growers in 2015 as a junior gardener. I was employed beginning in December 2015, in February 2016 I found out that I was pregnant, and resigned from my position later in May of 2016. While I was pregnant, I had some experiences while working at DC Growers which I now know to be traumatic.

During the time that I was working at DC Growers, I was exposed to a lot of environmental and workplace hazards that I should not have been exposed to as a pregnant person and reasonable accommodations should have been made for me within my rights of employment, even within cannabis cultivation. At the time, being my first pregnancy, I was unaware of many of these hazards and how to request reasonable accommodations without the threat of losing my job; this may have been common knowledge to the garden manager at the time.

Some of these hazards included cleaning the garden after the downstairs bloom room caught on fire, and the entire facility, including medicinal plants were covered in soot, hard, strenuous labor such as carrying five gallon buckets of water up/down stairs, dosing plants with harmful insecticides/pesticides that were not approved for medicinal plants, and working in the garden as it was being painted without proper ventilation. While completing these tasks, I was unaware of the effect that they would have on my body during and after pregnancy.

While working at DC Growers, I had to take two consecutive weeks off, due to severe lower back pain from carrying buckets of water. I could not walk comfortably for two weeks. I suffered from severe nausea up until the month I resigned. During this time, I spoke with my OB at

Johns Hopkins, who stated that he was unaware of the potential hazards of continuing to cultivate while pregnant and suggested I use my best judgment, which led me to resign from the position. I felt at the time, and still feel now, that harder tasks in the garden were assigned to me with the intention of making me quit, without having to fire me.

Although I was working at DCG for six months, I was not allowed to finish the junior gardener training that would have consisted of processing, less strenuous work, instead I was assigned remedial janitorial work around the garden.

In a male dominated industry, where very few women, especially childbearing women, have worked I did not have the resources, knowledge, or voice to advocate for myself. After my resignation, I began to further my education in cannabis and started advocating and supporting pregnant women and families who consume cannabis as a doula, childbirth educator, and cannabis consultant.

I was recently diagnosed with thyroid cancer and I felt I should tell my story. I'm writing this because I'm only now able to fully understand and articulate the traumatic experiences I endured while working at DC Growers while I was pregnant. Although what I shared here is not exhaustive, I hope it gives you an idea. More needs to be done to protect the rights and safety of pregnant women in the cultivation of medical cannabis, or working within the cannabis industry, and more needs to be done to advocate for the rights and needs of women and birthing people as it relates to cannabis consumption.

Thank you for taking the time to read this. I hope to work together with cannabis businesses to support the rights and needs of pregnant women and bring awareness to the many hazards within cannabis cultivation centers that may negatively impact people of childbearing age. You can learn more about my mission and the work I do to support pregnant women who consume cannabis, www.thecannabisdoula.org.

All the best,
Melanie Julion
www.thecannabisdoula.org

A Love Letter to Mars

April 22, 2020

Hey Mama's Baby,

My beautiful baby. You are my light. The apple of my eye. Your hugs
bring me joy, and peace, still. I love you like no other. Mars, your name
fits you—your fierce, strong, spirit…who eats nonstop. You are smart
and sensitive and love to cuddle with me and just like mommy, when you
don't get your way—you cry! Or just like daddy, you get mad!
Whatever it is, you are fierce.

I am proud of you.

I spend nights sometimes thinking about hugging you or kissing you.
You love books, and trucks, and paying with your brother.

Thank you for your spirit and energy.
And keeping me during this time.

You are finally two. Even though I've been saying you're two for some
time now. I am grateful for all the time we've had together.

Thank you for choosing me.

May 20, 2020

I will be thirty in seven days.

Every year, I am surprised to see the day and grateful for the opportunity. But thirty feels *different*.

While under normal situations, I suppose, there was going to be some grand celebration. I was actually supposed to be in LA with the boys, visiting my mom and sister, who we haven't seen in almost two years. What better way to celebrate. Due to the global pandemic, our flight was canceled back in April. We'd still be there. Our lives, completely different. Since these stay at home orders have been in place, and all of the hysteria of our society, I've had time to reflect on my life, and the lives of other families, our future, and how we can be self-sustaining as soon as possible. Especially when it comes to our medicine. Cannabis has been deemed essential. While at the same time, dispensaries are experiencing shortages and prices are steadily rising.

I rely on cannabis daily. I haven't been able to afford a consistent supply of RSO, so I've been trying my best to incorporate other natural remedies to support my healing, boosting my Endocannabinoid System and healing my thyroid. Even though I am not able to afford all of the herbs and supplements, or even the lifestyle changes that I need right now, I am working hard to get them because I deserve them.

Not having access to holistic remedies will not be a reason for me go against my beliefs about having surgery or using radiation and chemicals to treat cancer.

I'm excited to grow my own cannabis plants, and heal my own body, whenever that may be. I'll be supporting women with yoni steaming as a certified peristeam hydrotherapy facilitator and continuing to educate women and families on cannabis. In the midst of all of the chaos, I am exactly where I am supposed to be.

I hope to get a license to cultivate hemp, or medical marijuana, for myself and for a collective of women. I want to create a safe space for Black women to safely consume, talk about cannabis, and heal from trauma, and abuse infected on our wombs. I pray healing over our wombs.

I remember someone saying to me, and some other Black kids I was with, that a lot of us wouldn't make it to thirty. I just always assumed it would be me. Not Mitchell, or Jasmine, or Kristina, the best people I've ever known, still. I pray for our children's children. I pray that they won't live in fear of not living past 25.

I pray for the children whose heroes have died, and those whose heroes have died young.

May 21, 2020

On May 19th, our shining prince, our brother, Malcolm X would have been 95 years old. This year feels different. Since the release of the Netflix documentary, *Who Killed Malcolm X?* I can't help but question whether my ancestor is resting peacefully. There still must be justice in the matter of the assassination of Malcolm X. There is no longer any doubt that the US government and the members of the Nation of Islam conspired to create an environment where Malcolm X would be shot dead in front of his wife and children. They knew, and they lied, all these years. I pray for justice for Brother Malcolm, El-Malik-El hajj Shabazz. Our shining prince. I can never safely, and peacefully live in a country where Malcolm X, a human rights legend, could be gunned down a broad daylight, and his death never be investigated. Like Fred Hampton, Muammar al-Qaddafi, Patrice Lumumba, and many, many others. The lack of regard for Black bodies is no more evident than in the life of Malcolm X. I can never raise my children in this country, pretending like this never happened.

In Haiti, before the Haitian Revolution really jumped off, the first people to be killed by the revolting enslaved people, were the slave traitors. The enslaved Black people who had been so brainwashed that they were doing the work of the colonizer, slave masters, and white supremacists; the infiltrators. The people who were specifically placed in our community with the purpose of informing the slave master of anything that was going on in the slave quarters, amongst workers, in the church, in community organizations, in revolutionary movements. There has always been people amongst our own who do not work in our best interest and who specifically work against the Black community as a whole, while maintaining status amongst our community.

There are people like that among us today, celebrities, politicians, musicians, pastors, who only pretend to support Black people but are sleeping with the white supremacists. It's about class. Only a few Black people can rise to a status of wealth in this world without people feeling uncomfortable. So these few Black people who are at this level of wealth, class, and status, will do whatever they can to keep the rest of the Black community entertained, sleep, and unconscious. As long as we are entertained, we'll be quiet, we won't revolt. We'll forget. We'll get over it.

I used to think our society's focus on Black entertainment, music, and sports was to keep white people entertained. Now that all this shit is shut down due to COVID-19, I'm realizing all of this was set up to keep us distracted, busy, watching TV, watching sports, and going to work. All of the things that we busy ourselves with just to keep our ancestors from telling us to WAKE THE FUCK UP. Not only have we been thoroughly brainwashed into zombies, but we've been hypnotized beyond your wildest belief. These hypnotic suggestions are reinforced in our daily lives, in media, by companies, in advertising, to keep us in subordinate positions, because we believe them at a subconscious level.

We will never know our true history if we don't educate ourselves outside of the oppressors and the puppets that they use, who look like us but who are doing the work for them. We will never live our whole truths or our best lives by continuing to live a lie in this country. There is a reason the great Marcus Garvey, Malcolm X, and James Baldwin all spoke of the importance of internationalism and global African movements. There is a reason the greatest Black intellectuals and organizers and writers of our time were assassinated and or conspired against. We must wake up, and remember. Our Ancestors are fucking waiting, g.

You are not Black, don't you know?

You are melanin.

Language used to hypnotize and program the subconscious to make us inferior and act as such:

nigga/nigger,
bitch (black-witch), a curse
black (low-class, less than, poor), used with lowercase b

Environmental harm and genocide used to make us inferior:

Poor quality, unregulated, or contaminated cannabis
GMO foods
Heavy metals

Pesticides
Fracking
Pollutants in air
Poor water quality
Pollutants in water
Overpopulated areas
Poor living conditions and schools:
mold, roaches, old pipes, lead paint

Gemini New Moon | May 22, 2020

I welcome this day with gratitude. My best friend Kristina, made her transition on this day thirteen years ago. I sit with her. I sit with her spirit and everything she has taught me. I am better because of her And still have so much more to learn.

I look a suicide so much more differently, now than when I did at 16, or even at 25. I've probably come a lot closer to death myself. What a valuable lesson, and gift I have to carry your story within mine, my sister. We still have so far to go, but I'm grateful for everything you give me.

Jackson proposed to me last night, again.
I had to think about it.
This reoccurring proposal to marry and what that means,
what that looks like.

All I know is that I'm writing my book,
and loving my babies,
and all of this would not have been
had it not been for his love,
and for his courage.

The ancestors reminded me of compassion,
and forgiveness,
and mercy.
Have mercy.
Measure people right.
Compassion and loving is an ongoing
learning experience,
of letting go.

One writes out of one thing only—one's own experience. Everything depends on how relentlessly one forces from this experience the last drop, sweet or bitter, it can possibly give. This is the only real concern of the artist, to recreate out of the disorder of life that order which is art.

—James Baldwin

May 27th

I feel just like water.

I am one with all of the universe. I am truth, love, and peace. I am Sunday morning cuddles, and Wednesday morning love. I am a flower sprouting in springtime, leaves changing colors, falling to the ground in autumn. I am hot chocolate in a Chicago winter. I am the smell of a book store, and the pouring rain. I am like water for chocolate city. I am a sesh after a long week at work, or in the field. The first exhale. I am sacred space. I am an emerald. Like a stream returning to the ocean. I'm at home. I am grateful for my rebirth.

This journey has taught me strength, and the will to overcome seemingly unsurmountable obstacles and I pray that those who hear my story find peace in knowing that they too can overcome trauma and tragedy. I am grateful to be standing in truth and proud that I've never wavered in my pursuit for healing, for love, for peace, and for community, for all of us. You know, us melanated folks.

There is no doubt that the universe right now is filled with despair, death, and disease. Women and families are still suffering, as they were since before my journey began. But I dance, and celebrate life. I pray for healing on the hearts and wombs of Black women, may we continue on to birth the revolution.

I am sharing the joy of my ancestors all over the diaspora, by sharing my story and sharing lots, and lots, of cannabis.

May we all one day be free.

May 28, 2020

On the last night of my twenties, I went to sleep with an image of George Floyd being murdered in broad daylight by a Minneapolis police officer, his knee at the neck of limp, lifeless human being, a Black man who later died—while people watched and did nothing. This image was much like that of Eric Garner some years prior, and many others before and after him. Why do we fall victim to the Bystander effect and constantly watch our community be terrorized by pigs? Then, in the very next moment, people start asking "when will it end?"

When we realize we are living in an insane asylum where certain people feel that because of the color of their skin they are superior. So they use whatever methods of force, violence, and disease to depopulate and traumatize people to death. It's genocide that's happening here and until we realize that, the violence will persist. We are actively and passively allowing a genocide to occur in this country and we do nothing every time, every day, that a Black person is killed. This will only end when white women are able to come to terms with their own fear, and how their fear of Black men has caused irreparable harm to the lives of all Black men, women, and children, for generations.

From slavery, the murder of Emmett Till, and many others, due to white women's violence, the controlling of Black birthing bodies due to white women's jealousy and hatred, the sexual crimes committed against us at their will, the entire prohibition of our natural herbal medicine, cannabis, due to white people's fear related to the plant.

Now white women are silent. We see women, like the Karen in the park strangling the shit out of her dog just to shriek in horror to the police and lie on a Black man. We know women like them. Somehow, these women are still being protected as if a white woman lying on a Black person isn't enough for that person to be killed.

It should be of no surprise that on the day of my thirtieth birthday, I woke up to the news of riots sparking up in Minneapolis and other

Black cities.

People looting and burning down businesses.

A riot is the language of the unheard. Our ancestors will no longer allow for us to be quiet. The veil has been lifted from our eyes. Many of us would rather die in order to see our children's children live freely. Many of us have already died and more of us will have to die in order for the world to shift. I pray you be on the right side of justice. I pray you speak truth. I pray for the reparations, the freedom, that we are so due.

God gave Noah the rainbow sign, no more water,
The Fire Next Time.

Things I've Learned While Smoking Weed at 30

1. It is written. And you have the pen. If you want something, yes the entire universe will conspire to help you achieve it. But it takes hard work from you.
2. We have a decision to make in life and that is to remain complacent, comfortable and stagnant and accept what society deems a success or we can decide to expand our minds in a quest toward our own human revolution, to turn the poison into medicine.
3. Some of your friends will not make it to see thirty with you.
4. Read, profusely. Read so much that your ancestor's knowledge is enough to sustain you.
5. Be quiet.
6. Turn off the TV.
7. Your intuition is your most powerful weapon.
8. A Wise Woman once said, "not lift as you climb but rather, *leave no one behind*."
9. You are only as free as the people next to you.
10. Speak only truth, otherwise be quiet.
11. Be your own cheerleader.
12. Grow your own cannabis. Balance your Endocannabinoid System.
13. The revolution will not be televised, it will be a pain-free home birth.
14. The only one stopping you from being free is you.
15. You have the power to change poison into medicine. You are the alchemist.
16. Revolution is healing.

May 30, 2020

This week I celebrated my thirtieth birthday, in the midst of everything going on in this country. I wish there was a better time and place to celebrate such a thing. But, what a time to be alive. I can't help but think of the world that I was born into as a Black woman; a mother to two Black boys. I've literally grown up seeing Black bodies being killed on television since the LA riots in the early 90s; nothing has changed. I never thought that I would make it to thirty. My best friends have died, many people that I admire have all died or have been killed before the age of 30. That's the reality of our situation. I am grateful and humbled by the opportunity that I have to walk in my purpose and continue to do the work I've been called to do in supporting families and speaking my truth. But...I can't help but think, what are we doing here?

Our families are suffering. How can we talk about healthy birth practices in an environment that doesn't see us as human? How can we talk about reclaiming the use of our indigenous herbs, like cannabis, in a country that has strategically outlawed our natural remedies and our healers? This country was not set up for us to be well, for us to grow healthy children, for us to give birth without pain, for us to live freely, for us to prosper. We live in a country with people who are unable to see their hatred and racism as a mental disorder so they ignore it, make laws to enforce it, and remain silent or indifferent to our being murdered. Racism is a sickness; a disease of the blood. We live in a country where white women are raising their children who kill ours; and we continue supporting them— acting as if they are excused of any responsibility in the creation of a violent society that directly benefits them.

When I look at melanated people, I see myself. A part of my soul dies when I see another Black person unjustly killed. The trauma that we face just from seeing ourselves die on television our whole lives is trauma white children will never know. So I wonder, for white women, when you look at these people do you see yourself? Do you see yourself in the white woman in the park who was choking her dog in fear, or do you see yourself in every police officer that has killed a Black person, do you see yourself in white children who are shooting up schools? And if you don't, that is part of the problem. Because they are you. This is what you have given birth to.

413

Until "white" women realize that they are mothering children who are growing up to be racist, violent, abusive, killers— this cycle will not end. Until white women tell their sons, their brothers, their husbands and partners, dads, uncles, and friends to stop and own up to their own role in all of this, the cycle of racism and brutality against Black bodies will continue. Until white women can learn to mother a new culture in their community, one based on mutual love and respect for all living beings, nature, and melanated people, the world will not know peace. White women too, must heal their wombs. Heal your wombs that have given birth to generations of racism, death, and despair into this earth. Quiet your wombs so that the world will know peace. Let hate and fear no longer fill you. For the fate of your children, and mine, depends on you recognizing your own humanity. This is the world that you have birthed, and she is being burned down.

Questions for "white" women to consider:

- Where is the evidence-based information to support the racist, violent, behavior of your community?
- Why are you teaching your children that they are "white", and mine are "black"? What evidence do you have to support this claim?
- What responsibility have you had in maintaining racist practices, beliefs, and traditions in your family?
- What are you doing to heal your womb so that the racism in your blood is not passed on to future generations?
- How have you healed and released the hatred, racism, and disease that you have inherited as a "white" person?
- What have you done to address the karma you've inherited by those who came before you?
- What are you doing to address the mental disorder of racism and white supremacy?
- What have you done to redistribute the wealth, luxury, and lifestyle that you have been afforded due to your family's crimes against humanity, and crimes against Black people in this country and around the world?
- What have you done to redistribute the land that you have inherited from your family's involvement in the stealing of land from Black, native and indigenous sharecroppers and enslaved people?
- What have you done to redistribute the wealth and access that you

414

have been afforded because of colonization?

- What have you done to reconnect Black people to their ancestors that were enslaved or killed on your family's land?
- What have you done to reeducate "white" families on the accurate history of the world?
- What have you done to reeducate "white" children on the idea of race?
- What have you done to address the crimes of corporations and businesses who directly and indirectly harm Black people?
- What have you done to protect Black bodies from being killed, kidnapped, trafficked or used for sport?
- What have you done to protect the innocence of Black children?
- What have you done to protect the wombs of Black women against reproductive harm inflicted in hospitals?
- How are you supporting the families of people who have been affected by racism and white brutality?
- How have you addressed other women in their passive violence against Black families?
- How are you, and your fear, contributing to the over-policing of Black people?
- How have you accepted, and acted on, the propaganda that was created for you to fear and hate Black people?

Sharing a post on social media is not enough to excuse the responsibility that you have to not be racist in real life. Change your own community. The way you've been taught to mother and conduct business can no longer be off the backs of melanated women and families. The world is changing and they said, "it's time to be free."

I've used cannabis throughout my journey in battling racism and white supremacy, domestic violence, and the resulting anxiety, depression, and post-traumatic stress from the abuse and trauma that is inflicted on Black women daily. Cannabis has allowed me to heal. Cannabis has given me the power to create revolutionary causes and empower women and families in my community. It has allowed me to speak truth to power. I hope the information shared here will also give you the power, knowledge, and understanding you need in order to heal from the trauma in your own life and the negative experiences that we face as women, and the audacity to share your story.

June 2, 2020

When I was pregnant with my first baby, I had nightmares of Black folks rioting, chaos, and disaster. Fires everywhere. Buildings destroyed. People crying in the streets. I woke up sweating, crying, it was the worst shit ever. I remember it vividly. I was there, I felt it.

It looked like LA. The race riots in LA in the early 90s. I called my mom later that day and I asked her why I had memories of the race riots in LA. She said we were living in Long Beach at the time; then went on to describe stores that were burned down, the same stores I saw in my nightmare. Black women, birthing people, and families have generations and generations, layers and layers, of this kind of trauma not only related to police related violence, but also because of institutionalized racism in education, maternal health, real estate, cannabis, and every other industry we've helped cultivate.

The work I do through The Cannabis Doula is to support Black families, across the diaspora, who have been strategically secluded from accessing quality cannabis and cannabis education and care to support their consumption and cultivation; free of the stigma, bias, and discrimination in order to seek education in the first place.

There are plenty of white women and non-Black women who follow and support The Cannabis Doula, while at the same time Black women and families are still being criminalized for cannabis and completely left out of accessing the resources, education, and services that I provide.

If you support The Cannabis Doula, support The Cannabis Doula for *all women*, not just white women in your community.

June 5, 2020

We have a responsibility to ensure that Black families have access to quality cannabis medicine, cannabis education, support, and care to rebuild our communities from the war on drugs that ravaged our communities, destroyed our families, and turned our schools into pipelines to the prison industry.

We will not be silent when our families deserve more. We are the descendants of the enslaved African people who were stolen from their homeland to grow hemp on American plantations.

We are the descendants of the very people who were sharecroppers on their own land. Our people were traded globally with hemp seeds falling from their hair. We will not be sharecroppers in an industry built by our blood, an industry that thrives off of our culture.

It's blood on the leaves. Blood in the soil. And blood in the streets. Strange fruit, hanging from cannabis leaves. We see your silence and complicity. We will not be silent as our ancestral plants and traditions are colonized and Black people are still being criminalized for their consumption, babies being taken from their mothers.

When I graduated from undergrad, I marked my mortarboard with these revolutionary words of Assata Shakur, *"No one is going to give you the education you need to overthrow them."* My message to young people in this country remains the same. As young Black, Native, and Indigenous people in this country, we have an obligation and responsibility to fight for justice, revolution, and freedom for our people. They didn't tell you who your ancestors really were or why they were kidnapped and forced to live here. So you don't know who you are, or why you are here. All of this is by design. Get free. *We have nothing to lose but our chains.*

There is a reason cannabis education is not shared with us and is censored in our communities. There is a reason cannabis misinformation, propaganda, and fear-based, biased research is shared wildly in Black communities. There is a reason this information is being kept from Black midwives and birthing people. No one is going to give you the education you need to overthrow the pharmaceutical industry, the prison industry, the healthcare industry, or any other industry that profits off of the death of Black bodies. No one is going to give you the education you need to give birth freely and without pain, no one is going to give you the education you need to have healthy families. We must take it. We must own it. The future of our children depend on it. Our crowns have already been bought and paid for many, many times over. The time to heal our wombs is now.

Say her name. We demand justice for Breonna Taylor who was shot to death by police in her home, sleep in her bed on March 13th. We say her name, and the name of every other Black woman, trans woman, and ALL the children of Black women, young and old, killed by police violence and white brutality against Black families. There is a war on the wombs of Black women. Have you ever seen the look in the eyes of a Black mother who's child has been killed by police? Have you heard her screams? I have. I still do. Say their names. Happy Birthday, Breonna. We celebrate your life, and honor you sis.

Is your cannabis business complicit in the harm still being done to Black families and indigenous communities?

We demand cannabis reparations.

We demand equal access to cannabis education. We demand access to quality affordable cannabis. We demand cannabis tax revenue go to supporting families and communities negatively impacted by the war on drugs and cannabis prohibition. We demand justice for victims of the prison industry and police brutality. We demand equity and funding for Black cannabis entrepreneurs. We demand land. We will not be sharecroppers in an industry built on the backs and by the blood of our ancestors.

You are not exempt from your responsibility to advocate for the human rights of other people. We demand our human rights to consume and cultivate our traditional plants free of stigma, discrimination, and criminalization.

We will not be silenced.

Cannabis & The Black Woman

for Black Cannabis Magazine

Cannabis is the most consumed illicit drug by pregnant women, according to the World Health Organization, and apparently, most of these women are of low-income Black communities. Women across cultures have always consumed cannabis to support pregnancy related concerns, especially to treat symptoms related to nausea and vomiting, insomnia, pain, infection, and mental health concerns like anxiety, depression, and PTSD.

Since the earliest known uses of the cannabis plant, cannabis was used to support women and babies, especially by traditional doulas and Black Indigenous midwives before the advent of modern obstetrics and gynecology. Due to cannabis prohibition, the war on drugs, and racism related to cultivation and the cultural uses of the cannabis plant, much of this information has been suppressed and forgotten in Black and Indigenous communities in the United States. As Black women, and women all over the world, are starting to reclaim our traditional birth practices, without the influences of western medicine and white male doctors, we are once again reclaiming the use of the cannabis plant. We must do so safely, holistically, and with evidence-based information and care to support our cannabis consumption.

Doulas and midwives are an essential aspect of having a safe and natural birth. Like Black Grand Midwives, the original doulas were enslaved African women. In fact the word doula, is Greek for "female slave/servant," an obvious reflection of Black history in birth work. A doula is a pregnancy and birth professional who supports families during the childbearing years. Doulas provides mental, emotional, and physical support to birthing people during pregnancy, childbirth, and postpartum, especially providing advocacy, resources, and education. Doulas are birth coaches, birth assistants, and cheerleaders. We advocate for families, and often times help families in creating safe and empowering birthing experiences. Research has proven that having a doula will improve your birth outcome! Midwives are medical professionals with specialized medical training in supporting women's reproductive health concerns, including supporting natural birthing practices. The advent of western medicine allowed for the prohibition of traditional midwives and medicine women, healers, and herbal practitioners who used cannabis. Many midwives who used cannabis were outcast from their communities and persecuted as witches by the Catholic church, thus changing the way Black communities received medical care and related to African healing practices, especially during pregnancy and childbirth.

Through The Cannabis Doula, (www.thecannabisdoula.org) I provide holistic support services, education, and care to women and families who consume cannabis, especially during pregnancy, childbirth, and postpartum. Black and Indigenous communities and families that have been ravaged by the war on drugs and cannabis prohibition, deserve reparations and education, at the very least. Through Cannabis Doula Care Consultations and individualized cannabis care plans, families receive support to help them in safely and holistically consuming cannabis, making informed decisions, and talking to their doctors about medical marijuana. The *Holistic Cannabis Consumption: Pregnancy, Childbirth, & Postpartum online course* is a comprehensive childbirth education course focused on the traditional uses of cannabis during pregnancy, its historical uses in obstetrics, and cannabis-infused healing remedies for moms and babies emphasizing harm reduction, risk management, evidence-based information, and cannabis science.

As a doula, childbirth educator, and certified cannabis consultant and educator, I am really passionate about supporting women and families in safe consumption and shattering the stigma related to cannabis. If you are interested in learning more cannabis and pregnancy, yoni steaming, and other natural herbal remedies, schedule a consultation, enroll in a course. I look forward to sharing more of my personal journey using cannabis to support women's reproductive health and family wellness.

The second full moon of October has me in awe of the spirit of the universe. This month, *the women gathered*. We gathered at the Sacred Vibes Spiritual Herbalism Conference with Empress Karen Rose and we gathered again at the Reproductive Futurism Virtual Gathering with Doula Chronicles. We gathered to share in the dreams of our ancestors. We collectively dreamed of what a free Black future will look like. We set intentions. Bold, brave, majestic intentions. I presented on Cannabis Medicine in Pregnancy and Childbirth at the Reproductive Futurism Virtual Gathering, and I can't help but think of how it was my dream to connect with my doula sisters, to share the divine wisdom of the cannabis plant, only a few weeks prior at the Black Herbalists Convergence. The universe moves through me. Next week, I'm presenting on Cannabis to Support Perinatal Mental Health at the DMV Perinatal Mental Health Symposium.

This was my dream.

The story of Oshun continues to come up in sacred spaces. Black women are remembering, and removing ourselves from places that do not serve us. I'm powdering my nose on the moon. I recently began teaching parent education for an organization in DC, I'll also be facilitating workshops of healthy marijuana consumption for the staff and the community we serve. I'm pulling up to the table, ready to eat, teach, and feed my babies.

With the presidential election a few days from now, it seems like so much is on the line for Black women. At a time when the image of Breonna Taylor was glorified but her murders not charged for their crime; at a time when Black women's children are mis-educated killed, or imprisoned, at a time when Black mothers and babies are dying in childbirth and Black people are dying from COVID at drastic rates; at a time when we have a Black woman as a candidate for Vice President of the United States. I'm less than thrilled, to say the absolute least.

I wonder if Black Greek-Lettered Organizations were created just to keep us caught up in the idea that one of our own has made it; therefore so have we. I reject it. I pray we use our collective energy to rise above the oppression and lies being fed to us.

African youth on the continent are uprising against police brutality; and we still are too, as quiet as kept. I can't predict the future, but 2020 can't possibly end without a full-blown revolution. Perhaps, we too should burn our constitution and start over; or at least start with burning some cannabis.

Morning routine for a grounded and peaceful day
(in the midst of chaos and disorder) :

Rise & Shine:
Offer gratitude and set intentions
Wake and Bake with cannabis,
Crystal Sound Healing,
Tarot & Oracle
Yoga and Meditation,
Enjoy your favorite tea
Journal

A Black Girl's Guide to Holistic Cannabis Consumption

An Evidence-Based Practice

The mission of The Cannabis Doula is to support women, birthing people, and families who consume cannabis by providing family-centered, evidence-based cannabis education, holistic birth doula services, and support, including certified cannabis caregiver services.

The Cannabis Doula centers communities most impacted by cannabis prohibition and the war on drugs to provide safe access to quality cannabis and culturally-competent education in order to encourage holistic cannabis consumption.

The Cannabis Doula advocates for safe cannabis consumption, harm reduction and risk management, safe access, and equity in the form of reparations in the cannabis industry for Black and Indigenous women and families.

Our evidence-based practice is the integration of:

- **Clinical expertise and expert opinion:**
We use ancient, traditional, contemporary, and current research from experts in cannabis, neuroscience, obstetrics and gynecology, endocannabinology, nursing, and midwifery to support families in making informed decisions about cannabis.

- **External scientific evidence:**
Principles & Methods of Harm Reduction: Provides families with practical, safe methods to implement as they consume cannabis, if they choose, and tips to minimize harm and manage risks associated with cannabis use during pregnancy,

Bioecological Systems Theory & Cannabis Choosing Parents: Allows families to center the birthing person and create harmony in their environment to help support their use of cannabis as medicine.

Psychoeducational Model of Intervention: Combines evidence-based information with comfort measures, holistic doula support, and childbirth education to support the mind, body, and spirit of the birthing person.

- **Client/patient/caregiver perspectives:**

Since 2016, I've had the privilege of supporting cannabis consuming mothers in various ways in our community and online. I believe cannabis consuming mothers are experts in their experience, and I have crafted individualized care to support them.

Our Community

Women, cannabis moms, birthing people & their partners, caregivers, cannabis nurses & physicians who support cannabis and women's health. Through local and virtual events, classes, and services, we've connected with women and families who consume cannabis nationally and internationally. This is *Revolutionary Motherhood*.

- **Personal Expertise**

As a cannabis consuming parent, patient, and educator, I offer my first hand experience to families, which is invaluable for mothers seeking reassurance and community support.

The Cannabis Doula™ Approach

The Cannabis Doula provides support from a psychoeducational intervention model and harm reduction framework combining evidenced-based cannabis science with holistic childbirth education and family life education to assist families in making informed decisions on cannabis.

Evidence-Based Research

We incorporate endocannabinology, cannabis science and therapeutics, research, and education as well as evidence-based information on pregnancy, childbirth, postpartum, and parenting to support our community.

Holistic Comfort Measures

We use a holism framework to provide support to the whole person, mind, body, and spirit. We believe a balanced ECS + holistic cannabis consumption can support a natural pregnancy and a painless, blissful birth and postpartum experience.

Stigma Shattering Support

The Cannabis Doula provides support to create harmony between care providers and cannabis choosing families, and we are building an inclusive community for families who choose cannabis through Revolutionary Motherhood, our birth circle and support group, and advocacy through Birth Professionals for Medical Cannabis.

The Endocannabinoid System & The Female Body

Regulates homeostasis, mood, memory, immunity, and pain
To date, the ECS is comprised of endocannabinoids, like Anandamide and 2-AG, plus CB receptors, and other receptors in the body. CB1 receptors are located in the brain, spinal cord, and central nervous system. CB2 receptors are located in the peripheral organs, immune system, as well as the ovarian cortex, ovarian medulla, and ovarian follicles.

Regulates folliculogenesis, oocyte maturation, and ovarian endocrine secretion.
From our menstrual cycle, or the growth of human cells into a fetus, the ECS aids in proper functioning and managing related hormones

Modulates oviductal embryo transport, implantation, uterine decidualization and placentation. A healthy endocannabinoid-tone is important in maintaining a healthy fetus and placenta.

The Cannabis Plant

Cannabis is an annual, wind-pollinated, leaf-dropping herb that produces both flower and seeds. According to cannabis expert and neurologist, Dr. Ethan Russo, "Cannabis is the single most versatile herbal remedy, and the most useful plant on Earth. No other single plant contains as wide a range of medically active herbal constituents."

There are at least 554 identified compounds in the cannabis plant, including over 150 phytocannabinoids, like CBD and THC, 200 terpenes like myrcene and limonene, and flavonoids like cannaflavin A and B—which are unique to the cannabis plant. These compounds create an Entourage Effect by working synergistically to create a wide range of medicinal benefits.

Cannabis can best be understood by categorizing its mental and physical effects on the Broad to Narrow Leaf spectrum, from sedating to stimulating. On one end of the spectrum, Broad Leaf cannabis, commonly known as indica, is calming and sedating. On the other end is Narrow Leaf cannabis, often referred to as sativa, is stimulating and energizing. Medium Leaf cannabis plants provide a balanced effect, depending on the genetics, and are often referred to a hybrids. The various species of cannabis, hemp and marijuana, both range from sedating to stimulating, or calming to clearing, and can be used to create a unique, personalized medicine.

Cannabis has been grown all over the world and has been hybridized for hundreds of thousands of years. Scientists now believe cannabis to be polytypic, meaning that it contains multiple species. Within the Cannabaceae family, the main species of cannabis genus are cannabis indica, cannabis sativa, and cannabis rudaralis.

Strain names, like *LA Chocolat* and *Acapulco Gold*, are used to identify various cultivars of hemp and marijuana. However, relying on strain names alone may not be a sufficient way to distinguish the effects of the flower because the effects and quality of cannabis can change based on grow method, location, skill of grower, products used, lights, etc.

Hemp
cannabis sativa ssp. sativa

- Mildly-psychoactive, non-euphoric, non-hallucenagenic
- Legally contains less than 0.3% of THC
- CBD-Rich variety, also used for grain and fiber
- 2018 Farm Bill legalized Hemp in all 50 states under certain regulations
- Spectrum of effects range from calm (Broad Leaf Hemp) to clearing (Narrow Leaf Hemp)

Marijuana
cannabis indica ssp. afganica,
cannabis indica ssp. indica, etc.

- Psychoactive, euphoric "high"

- Hallucinogenic properties due to high THC levels
- Many varieties of marijuana have been bred specifically to produce high levels of THC, and lower levels of CBD, and other cannabinoids
- States and countries are moving to decriminalize, legalize, and regulate medical and recreational marijuana
- Spectrum of effects range from sedative (Broad Leaf Marijuana) to stimulating (Narrow Leaf Marijuana)

Tip from The Cannabis Doula:
grow your own
or know your grower

The Cannabis Doula™ Philosophy on Pregnancy and Birth

Our goal is to empower childbearing people to be confident, trust in their innate ability to give birth naturally, and make informed decisions about interventions during pregnancy, childbirth, and postpartum---from breastfeeding, parenting, through early childhood, including the use of cannabis and other medications.

Pregnancy is a life changing spiritual journey, a mind-body-spirit transformation, and rites of passage, that prepares people for parenthood and the birth of a family. Culturally-competent family support and education is necessary for the health and wellness of families.

Why Cannabis and Birthwork?

Many moms consume cannabis, with very little education and support. In fact, cannabis is the most consumed "illicit drug" by pregnant women, according to The World Health Organization and ACOG, the American College of Obstetricians and Gynecologists. As more and more pregnant women are openly praising the healing properties of cannabis for common pregnancy/postpartum concerns, even pain in childbirth, and more research is being done to support the use of cannabis during pregnancy, we must recognize cannabis as a potential alternative to many dangerous interventions and pharmaceuticals during pregnancy, childbirth, and the postpartum period, and how safe, healthy cannabis consumption can benefit families, with little to no side effects.

Cannabis, consumed in various methods, can address many of the health concerns that women have throughout our lifetimes including nausea during pregnancy, pain during birth, postpartum hemorrhage and depression, painful periods, pain during sex, vaginal dryness, symptoms related to PCOS, endometriosis, breast cancer, fibromyalgia, and more.

Choosing cannabis is a healthcare decision and a birth choice for all families, and all families deserve access to cannabis education, support, and care to support the safe use of medical cannabis before, during, and after pregnancy. The Cannabis Doula provides a variety of services and family-centered education including holistic doula services, cannabis caregiver services (cultivation and medicine crafting), cannabis-infused yoni steaming, sound healing, meditation, yoga, and sacred cannabis events and seshs.

Ancient & Traditional Cannabis Use for Women's Health

Africa
Ancient Egypt / Continental Africa
African Healing Practices
smsm-t, ganga, banga used in all forms; Administered orally, rectally, vaginally, on the skin, in the eyes, and by fumigation. To support childbirth and depression; method of smoking in childbirth originated here. Cannabis was said to be associated with the female Pharaohs and goddess Seshat. A well-known preparation was cannabis "ground with honey and introduced in vagina."

Iran
Ancient Mesopotamia / Persia
Azallû, banga used for difficult childbirth and staying the menses & various female ailments. Hemp flower, roots, and seeds mixed were often with beer and other herbs for tinctures. The original idea of pharmacies were created here using cannabis as medicine by highly skilled Arabian physicians.

China
Ancient / Traditional Chinese Medicine
Hemp seeds widely used to treat a variety of conditions from breastfeeding problems to nourishing the blood. Cannabis is commonly used to balance deficiencies in yin.

India
Southeast Asia
Ayurvedic Medicine
Bhang tea, hashish balls, dishes containing hashish are used for tantric, and as an aphrodisiac, to treat pain, hemorrhage, and other common conditions of women and children.

Europe
Ancient Greek / Rome
haenep, or hemp, used for swelling, sore breast and to support difficult childbirth.

Americas
North and South American Indigenous and Slave traditions, U.S. Pharmacopoeia
Used underground with different names to disguise its use, weed, marijuana, Rosa Maria. Hemp was used for dysmenorrhea, menopause, menorrhagia, labor, uterine cancer, uterine disorders, pain, melancholia, infant colic, hemorrhage.

African Healing Traditions
A Brief African History

Cannabis, also known as dagga, or diamba, across Sub-Saharan Africa; was commonly used to fight malaria, black water fever, as an aesthetic during childbirth, and a cure for asthma. The ethnobotany of cannabis included pipe smoking, a practice invented and perfected in Africa. Ground cannabis seed is still sometimes used as baby food across many areas and tribal practices on the continent.

There is conflicting accounts on whether cannabis spread with Islam or trade into Africa, or out of Sub-Sahara Africa to Egypt, Mesopotamia and to the rest of the world via trade. Much of the history of cannabis in Africa has been either suppressed, hidden, or orally told and intentionally distorted, but it now being reclaimed.

The African innovation of smoking the cannabis plant initiated the global practice of smoking marijuana, which changes the drug pharmacologically. Africans developed diverse cultures of cannabis use, including African practices that circulated widely in the Caribbean and South and North Americas via slave trading. The term marijuana was later used by indigenous Mexicans to disguise the use of the sacred plant from Spanish colonizers and the catholic religion.

Cannabis was also commonly used by Tswana, Zulu, Sotho, and Swazi people at that time. During British rule in the 1800s, Indian indentured servants living in South Africa widely used cannabis. Anthropologists across central and east Africa have noted traditional cannabis use among native tribes. However, by the 1920s, cannabis was outlawed across most of the continent. African people have resisted cannabis prohibition in the attempt to preserve their traditional uses of the plant. Underground cannabis production remains economically significant despite the dangers of cultivation and consumption.

Hemp traveled to the New World via the Trans-Atlantic Slave Trade, and was already cultivated and used in many Native American traditions. Native Americans used cannabis as medicine for treating inflammation and other issues, and they also used it in ceremonial peace practices. As a way to seal a peace treaty, opposing sides were said to have smoked cannabis together using a Native American peace pipe. However, British colonizers were sent with direct orders to grow hemp, especially in states in Kentucky, Missouri, Illinois and Florida. British colonizers were compelled by law to grow hemp, and many of them considered it their patriotic duty. In order to meet the demand, they implemented the use of plantation style slave labor. The use of free labor by enslaved African people grew both the cotton industry, and the hemp industry, that was needed for the bagging and roping necessary for mass cotton production.

Africans arrived in North America as explorers, traders, servants, and some enslaved around the 16th century. It was assessed that it took three enslaved people to manage every 50 acres and the most skilled hemp cultivators, enslaved Black men, were highly sough after. Without slavery the hemp industry would not have operated.

Seeds and traditions traveled with enslaved people, who used cannabis as medicine, and to smoke for spiritual purposes. Africans often grew their own for cannabis for recreational use, encouraged by Plantation owners, who used cannabis to keep enslaved people "happy" or in subordinate positions.

Kentuckians, and quite possibly many other white people and slave plantation owners, referred to hemp as a *nigger crop*, believing that no one understood the eccentricities of cannabis as well or with such expertise in handling the plant as "the Negro."

Cannabis in Western Medicine:
Early Obstetrics & Gynecology and Midwifery

Cannabis was used in U.S. pharmacology from the 1800s - 1940s
Eumetra, a cannabis preparation, considered the ideal analgesic for uterine irritation. Dysmenine, a cannabis tincture for menstrual cramps was popularly used, including other tonics, capsules, and infant syrups with cannabis were also widely used as homeopathic medicine. These are just some examples of the many cannabis medicine options available during the height of cannabis medicine. Other products included hashish candy, asthma inhalers, and various tonics and tinctures used for depression and infant colic. Pharmaceutical giant, Pfizer, was known as Park-Davis Co. during this time and manufactured some of the leading cannabis medicines.

Cannabis was often associated with witchcraft,
traditional healers, and Black Midwives
Cannabis has always been used by African people for spiritual purposes; this was associated with evil and disliked by the pope/ Christian religion. Cannabis use in childbirth survived the Middle Passage, where enslaved women skilled in herbs and midwifery often used cannabis and other herbal preparations on Black and white women.

J. Marion Sims experimented on Enslaved Black Women using hemp
J. Marion Sims used hemp string in the attempt to perfect his suture technique on an enslaved Black woman, without the use anesthetic. Af-

ter failing multiples times with hemp string, on his 30th attempt, using metallic sutures, he was successful in what would become his well-known vesico-vaginal fistula surgery. With no regard to his many victims, Black women and their babies, he is regarded to many as the Father of Gynecology and his methods are still practiced.

Many early medicine men experimented with the use of cannabis and other herbal remedies in an attempt to replicate the traditional herbal recipes of Black midwives. The use of cannabis and other herbs were not just used on enslaved women. White women, Native American women, and Black women relied on the used of herbal medicine for common female ailments and readily shared and exchanged remedies and knowledge across cultures. Many women of the time believed, as many still do, that women's care was best treated with-woman, the traditional midwife.

Cannabis & Pregnancy

Cannabis can provide direct and indirect relief to common pregnancy concerns and has been traditionally used to support women and birthing people.

Cannabis can be used to aid in the following pregnancy related concerns: nausea, vomiting, pain, anxiety, depression, PTSD, mood imbalances, GI issues, constipation, diarrhea , heartburn, asthma, gestational diabetes, eczema; severe itching, low libido, dry skin, sleep disturbances, incontinence, bladder issues, and to stimulate or suppress appetite.

Why Women Choose Cannabis During Pregnancy

First Trimester
Nausea/vomiting, anxiety, depression, regular/new cannabis consumers, natural pregnancy, stimulate appetite, mood imbalances

Second Trimester
Discomfort, nausea/vomiting, hemorrhoids, natural and traditional alternative, instinctual, cultural use

Third Trimester
Fear, anxiety, pain/discomfort, nausea/vomiting, appetite stimulant, bowels, energy, sleep disturbances

Hyperemesis Gravidarum

A common pregnancy complication characterized by severe nausea, vomiting, weight loss, and dehydration. In severe cases, HG can cause birthing people to terminate a pregnancy, or lead to severe complications for mother and baby. Many people have severe nausea during pregnancy, and find very little relief from pharmaceutical drugs or other natural remedies.

How cannabis can support HG:

The Endocannabinoid System is involved in the control of nausea/vomiting and the visceral sensation.

Cannabis has the ability to treat symptoms of inflammation and functional disorders of the GI tract that can lead to nausea/vomiting due to anti-nausea, antiemetic properties of cannabinoids and terpenes.

CBD in Pregnancy, Childbirth, & Postpartum

Non-Euphoric
CBD-dominant, low-THC strains of cannabis provide medical benefits, support, and relief, without the mind altering high of THC.

Safe for Mom and Baby
Anxiolytic, anti-depressive, nonaddictive, non-convulsive, pain relieving, and tumor killing properties; mildly psychoactive; enhances efficacy of THC, but reduces high

High CBD strains
Supports a wide range of conditions and illnesses: anxiety, depression, spasms, pediatric seizures, colic, lactation issues, etc.

Cannabis Use to Support
Perinatal Mental Health & Wellness

Many of the earliest uses for cannabis in treating women was for mental health, and what many doctors at the time referred to as an unknown female ailment, or uterus hysteria (hysteria of the uterus), and other conditions of the womb that caused depression or anxiety. Birthing people have resorted to the use of cannabis for depression and anxiety during pregnancy and for treating and preventing postpartum depression.

Perinatal & Postpartum Depression

Cannabis is an alternative to antidepressants, used throughout history, to stimulate the ECS and speed up the growth and development of nervous tissue with little side effects. CBD decreases risk of suicide, and reduces the use and abuse of alcohol, cigarettes, opioids, meth, etc.

Treating depression/ PPD is complex. CBD activates 5HT1A Serotonin Receptors and elevates dopamine levels to improve mood and anxiety, and Endocannabinoid Deficiency related to drops in estrogen 3-4 days postpartum. CBD can also help to manage the increase in inflammation during childbirth that may be linked to postpartum depression.

Cannabis treatment options for perinatal/postpartum depression may include CBD, CBD+THC, 1:1, 10:1; and varies based on the birthing person.

Anxiety

The ECS appears to play an important role in responses to stress and anxiety. THC and CBD, appear to have differing effects with regard to anxiety. Pure THC appears to decrease anxiety at lower doses. CBD appears to decrease anxiety at all doses that have been tested. THC / Narrow Leaf cannabis plants can exasperate anxiety, trigger paranoia. Therefore, cannabis treatment options for anxiety may be CBD- Dominant strains with very low doses of THC, if at all.

Addressing Fear and Anxiety Related to Childbirth

The true elephant in the birth room. The topic that so many are afraid to discuss, but will readily divulge to scare a first time mom. That is, the pain associated with childbirth. Some researchers believe that pain in childbirth is just a mental programming of all the things we've seen and heard about childbirth in the media. Others believe that pain is a vital, necessary part of the birthing process, to inform the birthing person to seek shelter or change positions to help with the descent of the fetus. Others believe that pain during childbirth is women's punishment to bare. Whatever your belief, many women experience some anxiety as it relates to childbirth, losing control, or the fear of the unknown. In South Africa, doctors reported giving dagga to women to help them be brave so that they don't feel pain. Cannabis use may be able to help address underlying fears that we have about giving birth and help us to release them so that we can achieve a healthier, safer birthing.

Post-Traumatic Stress Disorder (PTSD)

CBD and THC are capable of helping people relieve symptoms related to PTSD by improving the ECS' mediation of essential functions including memory consolidation and retrieval. By activating CB1 and CB2 receptors, cannabinoids appear to prompt the system to produce Anandamide, the bliss molecule, helps promote happiness, pleasure, and memory.

Birth Trauma

People with PTSD have much lower levels of anandamide. PTSD may develop following a traumatic birth, related to pain, childhood/sexual trauma, birth experience, hospital care, racism.

Inhalation of cannabis may be most effective in treating immediate concerns, CBD+THC.

Cannabis as Pain Management

Cannabis addresses these three physical causes of pain in childbirth: Visceral, Somatic, and Nerve Compression. Cannabis addresses nociceptive pain by reducing pain signals at the source of the discomfort by blocking the inflammatory process and the signals they elicit.

Cannabis addresses our mental perception of pain, the fear and anxiety that causes pain. Cannabinoids may increase pain thresholds but do not appear to reduce the intensity of pain already felt. They also appear to help people handle more pain; which is especially useful for mothers as they are able to be present in childbirth.

Cannabinoids appear to make pain feel less unpleasant and more tolerable, which implies cannabinoids are influencing the affective component of pain rather than the sensory aspect.

Cannabis Analgesic for Childbirth

An analgesic is a pain-relieving drug often categorized as NSAIDS (Non-Steroidal Anti- Inflammatory Drugs) and opioids (narcotics). These drugs are usually prescribed based on the severity of pain, according to the World Health Organization.

Analgesics are routinely prescribed to pregnant women administered during childbirth, and prescribed during postpartum to nursing mothers, regardless of the harmful side effects, risks to mom/baby, and the risk of NAS in the newborn. We believe that due to the harmful risks associated with NSAIDS and opioid use in pregnant and nursing women, and the high risks of abuse and addiction, cannabis is the best and safest possible alternative in supporting women experiencing pain during pregnancy, childbirth, and postpartum.

> Cannabis Analgesia provides a good example of its potential as a harm reduction medication. Innumerable chronic pain patients have found it difficult to find a balance between managing their pain and being able to function in daily life. Opiates are frequently used for management of severe pain, however they sometimes leave the patient feeling "drugged" and come with the risk of overdose and side effects such as constipation, nausea, and vomiting. Increasingly, patients are acting on the advice of others and are trying cannabis as an analgesic...The introduction of cannabis into pain management regimens has been very helpful. Most patients report a significant reduction in the use of opioids of the need them on occasion for acute ex- dependence. Cannabis is an effective antiemetic, and is not constipating. In summary, many chronic pain

438

patients who use cannabis report that they feel better, experience fewer untoward side effects, and are able to reduce their use of opioids and other medications, and are thereby able to eliminate additional side effects that many accompany those medications as well as the added risks from drug interactions. *(Cannabis and Harm Reduction: A Nursing Perspective, Mary Lynn Mathre. Women and Cannabis: Medicine, Science, and Sociology, 2002)*

Common medications used for treating pain in pregnant and nursing people:

Mild-to moderate pain:
NSAIDS (anti-inflammatory, pain/fever reducer) Motrin, ibuprofen, Advil, Aspirin
Acetaminophen: (pain reliever/fever reducer) Tylenol, Midol

Moderate to severe pain:
Low-dose opioids, opiates, narcotics
Codeine (Tylenol 3), dihydocodeine, tramadol

Severe pain:
High-dose opioids, opiates, narcotics
Oxycodone (OxyContin), morphine (Demerol), Fentanyl, Percocet, Vicodin

Cannabis contains natural analgesic properties and in its various forms can be administered to address mild, moderate, and severe pain and inflammation with less harmful effects than those listed above.

In addressing pregnant people who are addicted to pain killers, or synthetic opioids (heroin, meth): CBD can help treat issues of addictions, as an analgesia cannabis can manage and treat the sources of pain, and provide comfort to symptoms. It is nonaddictive, and shows no harmful effects to moms or baby, in addition it aids in homeostasis.

In addressing pregnant people during childbirth: Cannabis analgesia provides a safer alternative to opioids used to as pain management in childbirth. Cannabis addresses pain receptors in the pain pathway and the categories of pain throughout the stages and phases of childbirth. Cannabis is especially useful during the stages and phases of birth because it provides support to the mind, body, and spirit, helps bring the body back into homeostasis (adaptation) between contractions and after birth, and helps build our sensation threshold.

Benefits of Cannabis in Childbirth

- THC releases oxytocin, the love hormone!
- THC and CBD can be used to increase the speed of labor.
- THC increases the body's response to endorphins, our natural painkillers, and increases anandamide, our internal bliss molecule.
- Direct relief through cannabinoid receptors in the uterus
- Cannabis use during childbirth does not cause withdrawal symptoms in infants and does not interfere with breastfeeding.
- Variety of consumption methods.
- THC disrupts pain pathway in the brain causing us to perceive pain as less severe
- Supports adaptation between birthing waves by helping to balance the ECS.

Naturally Support the Endocannabinoid System

- *Maintain Balanced Nutrition:* Healthy Diet, Vitamins & Nutrients, High Water Intake
- *Incorporate Cannabimimetic Practices:* Activities that mimetic the effects of cannabinoids in supporting our body's ECS:

Exercise
Yoga
Meditation
Sleep
Stress Management
Chiropractic care
Acupuncture
Aromatherapy
Social Engagements
Unstructured play time: Freedom
Osteopathic Manipulation (OMT)
Massage
Breathing exercises
Any voluntary and enjoyable exercise

- *Plants and herbs that engage the Endocannabinoid System:* Echinacea, Electric daisy, Liverwort, Dark Cacao, Black Pepper, Turmeric

- *Add essential fatty acids to your diet:* Hemp seeds, flax seeds, chia seeds, eggs, walnuts

- *Consume organic foods:* avoid storing food in plastic and be mindful of environmental toxins present in food and water.

- *Detox, often.* Cleanse the blood of heavy metals and harmful substances that lead to disease and illness.

- *Alcohol impairs ECS.* Avoid consuming cannabis with alcohol, as with recreation, or abuse. Consume cannabis with intent for the most medicinal benefit.

Cannabis & Family Wellness
Preventative care and daily use for the whole family

Cannabis in various forms and methods of consumption can be used to support the whole family, from children and teens to elders. Cannabis can be used as a preventative health aid, for daily use, and acute care.

- Reduces inflammation of the joints and tissues that can occur due to a number of chronic diseases including chronic pain
- Cancer prevention; kills, prevents growth of cancerous cells
- Slows Aging; stops the increasing the progress of Alzheimer's disease
- Heart disease; hypertension, obesity
- Digestion; Leaky gut, gas
- Strong bones, Bone protection: CB1 receptors found in the bones, and elsewhere in the body, respond positively to the use of cannabis. The cannabinoids then work to thicken and strengthen bones.

Learn more about the Cannabis & Family wellness course and workshop, visit www.thecannabisdoula.com.

Traditional Medicine in Preparation for Childbirth

Traditional Medicine is a combination of techniques, theories, modalities, and medical systems that aren't usually taught at most western medical schools or practiced in U.S. Hospitals. They are "alternative" to today's conventional, biomedical health care but are natural, ancient and traditional practices, all of which can be safely incorporated for a happy, healthy, and holistic pregnancy, childbirth, and postpartum.

We believe in the holistic approach to pregnancy and childbirth and support birthing people in incorporating a variety of traditional practices to promote and achieve a natural childbirth.

Ayurvedic Medicine: aromas, gems, herbs, lifestyles, massage, meditation, music, nutrition, purification, rejuvenation and yoga.

Chiropractic Science (American medicinal approach): When the spine is misaligned, problems occur. Drugless, Non-invasive. Adjusts, manipulates body. Decrease labor time.

Environmental Medicine: Cause/Effect of patients environment and illness. Household cleaners, cosmetics, food allergies or sensitivities.

Herbal Medicine: Originally all medicine was herbal, Wise Women (traditional midwives) used herbs traditionally to support pregnancy and birth.

Homeopathic Medicine: Non-addictive natural medicines, sold in health stores, essential in pregnancy, childbirth, postpartum, and for babies.

Naturopathic Medicine: Combines alternative medicine, therapeutic techniques with modern medicine and biochemistry.

Chinese Herbal Medicine: Uses roots, barks, flowers, seeds, leaves, fruit, branches to treat problem, strengthen immune system, maintain health.

Holistic Medicine: (This is our Happy place!) Combines a variety of practices to treat the whole person. Mind, body, spirit, their lifestyle, environment and family. Socio-biological. Holism is the framework used to build the goals, objectives, and learning in the *Holistic Cannabis Consumption: Pregnancy Childbirth and Postpartum course* and Happy Brown Baby Holistic Childbirth Education classes. CNMs, childbirth educators, nurses, physicians, and other health care professional often advocate for the holistic approach. The goal in Holistic Childbirth is facilitation rather than control of the birthing process.

Osteopathy: A hands-on approach that uses touch to help the body move efficiently. Osteopathic manipulation and massage is great for lower back pain during pregnancy.

Crystal and Gemstone Healing: Balances and heals chakras and related illnesses and blockages.

Light Therapy: Helps treat depression, seasonal affective disorder in pregnant people.

Energy/Body work: Hypnotherapy, Reiki, Dance Therapy, reflexology. The "laying on of hands" was used by Black traditional midwives.

Nutrition Science: *Let thy food be thy medicine.* Balanced Diet, Vitamins/Minerals.

Diet and Nutrition is especially important; it is essential in maintaining a healthy pregnancy, having a pleasant birth experience and for postpartum wellness. The utmost consideration should be made when choosing foods to eat during pregnancy. Eat foods that are organic, clean (free of pesticides, preservatives, etc.), and appealing to mom and baby. It's okay to appease pregnancy cravings, in moderation and with understanding of why the craving exists.

Usually when we crave something during pregnancy, it's our body's way of telling us we need a particular nutrient, vitamin, or sustenance that that particular food can provide.

Important Vitamins/ Nutrients for a healthy Pregnancy, Childbirth, and Postpartum

- **Folate** *(Prevent Birth Defects):* Fruit/vegetables, beans, leafy greens, cereals. Increase Folate/ Folic Acid if consuming THC during pregnancy as THC use can inhibit the uptake of folic acid.
- **Iron** *(Prevent Anemia)*: Green leafy vegetables, beans, cereals
- **Calcium** *(Strengthen Bones):* Broccoli, kale, dairy, fruit juices, cereals
- **Vitamin D** *(Promotes Bone Growth):* Fatty fish, juice, milk, eggs, sunshine
- **Protein** *(Promotes Growth):* Lean meat, poultry, fish, eggs, beans, nuts, seeds, soy
- **Vitamin C** *(Protects Tissue, Iron Absorption)*: Fruit/vegetables, Oranges, Peaches, Mango, Guava, strawberries, peppers, potatoes, papaya
- **Vitamin A** *(Supports Bones and Teeth)*: green and yellow fruit/vegetables, potatoes, pumpkin, carrots, eggs, milk
- **B- Vitamins** *(Thiamin, Riboflavin, Niacin, Pyridoxine prromotes energy and general health of hair, skin, and eyes):* Avocado, banana, sweet potato, high protein foods, meats, beans, nuts/seeds, wheat, oat, broccoli, cabbage
- **Zinc** *(Produces insulin/enzymes):* Red meats, poultry, beans, nuts, dairy, grains, cereals

It is also important to eat a variety of foods that are of cultural importance to the birthing family during pregnancy and postpartum. Remember: It is not the care provider's credentials but rather their philosophy that determine their preference for a physiological, natural, or holistic approach to birth.

Is Cannabis Safe During Pregnancy?

Cannabis is an alternative health aid traditionally used by women in various cultures around the world to support women in pregnancy, childbirth, and postpartum. Using positive language when talking about cannabis use during pregnancy can help to minimize harm and stigma related to cannabis use.

The Cannabis Doula integrates cannabis education, family life education, and childbirth education to help support families as they answer the question, "Is cannabis safe during pregnancy?" and implement methods of harm reduction and risk management to incorporate strategies for safe cannabis consumption, or cessation.

The *Holistic Cannabis Consumption: Pregnancy, Childbirth, and Postpartum* course and workshop focuses on the traditional uses of cannabis for women's health, its historical uses in obstetrics, and the use of cannabis-infused remedies for moms and babies during pregnancy and beyond. In the course, we dissect current research, cannabis laws and regulations, and Shatter The Stigma associated with cannabis use during pregnancy. Course participants receive support from a psychoeducational intervention model, and harm reduction framework, combining evidence-based information, childbirth education, family life education and cannabis science to assist families in making informed decisions on cannabis.

The course is intended to provide support for birthing people and families, especially those interested in learning how to make informed decisions about cannabis, supported by evidence-based information and cannabis science. This course is also great for doulas, childbirth educators, and other birthworkers including midwives and OB-GYNs, cannabis educators, caregivers, cannabis industry professionals such as dispensary agents and patient care specialists. To learn more and enroll, visit www.thecannabisdoula.org.

Risks Often Associated With Cannabis Use in Pregnancy

Current research on cannabis and pregnancy does not take into account confounding factors (such as tobacco, alcohol consumption, poor prenatal care) or other risk factors that influenced the following outcomes:
• Disruption of endogenous cannabinoids
• Pre-Term Birth
• Low Birth Weight/ Small for Gestational Age
• Adverse Neonatal Outcomes
• Higher-pitched cries
• Decreased attention, academic abilities, and cognitive functioning in adolescence
• Child Protective Services
Current research does not take into account type of cannabis used, method of consumption, frequency of use, and other measures to accurately determine risks.

The Cannabis Doula
S.A.F.E. Strategies for Consuming Cannabis:

To assist families in making an informed decision about cannabis use during pregnancy, I encourage families to create a S.A.F.E. Zone that centers the birthing person, providing support, education, and care for a healthy pregnancy. Always determine if your cannabis is safe to consume before consuming your cannabis flower or product.

S- Source and Smell: Is the source of this cannabis safe, trusted, reliable? Is the smell attractive, pungent, fresh/floral?

A- Attractive Attributes: Is the cannabis green, vibrant, and sticky with full buds and no seeds?

F- Feelings of Fear: How do I feel about consuming cannabis? How does my support and care team feel? What fears do I need to heal in order to use cannabis intentionally?

E- Effects / Energy: How do I feel after using cannabis? Record how you feel each time you consume cannabis to help track and manage your use.

Maximize your S.A.F.E. Zone

Create a SAFE Zone that can't be permeated with cannabis mis-information, propaganda, and stigma and be intentional with your cannabis use. You can also use the following affirmations to support you on your journey.

1. Visualize your S.A.F.E. Zone that can't be permeated with cannabis propaganda, misinformation, or stigma. (If you need help with this, book a Cannabis Doula Care Consultation!)
2. Set your intention.
3. Interpene cannabis for its quality
4. Assess your method of consumption (and your source!)

The Cannabis Doula
Pregnancy & Birth Affirmations

I am happy,
my baby is healthy,
we are healthy and whole
(Recite while consuming cannabis to help lessen fear/anxiety as
you inhale and exhale)

Healthy Mama,
Happy Baby,
Healthy ECS

Harm Reduction
Principles and Methods to support cannabis consuming families

Harm Reduction is of the upmost importance for expectant and nursing mothers and children, elders, and people with preexisting health conditions.

The Cannabis Doula uses harm reduction to incorporate a spectrum of strategies/interventions, from our S.A.F.E. Strategies for Consuming Cannabis and tracking and managing use, to examining cannabis quality and cessation to meet cannabis moms, or cannabis choosing families where they are, addressing the conditions of and for their cannabis use along with the quality of the cannabis itself.

The Cannabis Doula Principles of Harm Reduction

Harm reduction, as defined by the Harm Reduction Coalition, is a set of practical strategies and ideas aimed at reducing negative consequences associated with drug use, or a specific activity. Harm Reduction is also a movement for social justice built on a belief in, and respect for, the rights of people who use alternative substances.

The Cannabis Doula™ considers the following Principles of Harm Reduction central in supporting women and families who choose to consume cannabis:

- Licit and illicit cannabis consumption is part of our world, our society, and our culture and therefore we choose to work to minimize any potential harmful effects or misinformation rather than ignore or condemn the use of cannabis (marijuana, hemp, CBD, THC, etc.)
- Cannabis is a complex and multi-faceted plant and its use encompasses a continuum of behaviors from sacred use to abuse and misuse to total abstinence, and we acknowledge that some methods of consuming cannabis may be safer than others.
- The well-being and quality of the individual, family, and community life is the criteria for successful interventions and policies, not necessarily cessation of cannabis use.
- We demand non-judgmental, non-coercive provisions of birth and family support services and resources to families of color who use cannabis and the communities in which they live in order to assist them in becoming informed cannabis consumers.
- The Cannabis Doula™ urges communities to work together to Shatter The Stigma associated with cannabis use during pregnancy and any policies that may have resulted from the stigma and led to discriminatory practices such as nonconsensual drug testing of women and babies at childbirth, separating mother from child, etc.
- The Cannabis Doula™ moves to ensure that Black women and birthing families who use cannabis, and have traditionally and historically consumed cannabis, routinely have a real voice in the creation of programs and policies designed to serve them.
- Birthing people themselves are the primary agents in reducing the harms of their cannabis consumption, and we seek to empower birth professionals to share information and support families in strategies which meet the conditions of their cannabis use.
- We recognize that the realities of racism, class, poverty, social stigma and isolation, past trauma, sex-based discrimination and other social inequalities—including the War on Drugs, cannabis propaganda and misinformation, affect both people's vulnerability to and capacity for effectively seeking cannabis education and care to reduce harm.

The Cannabis Doula does not attempt to minimize or ignore the real and tragic harm and danger caused by the War on Drugs and cannabis prohibition to Black, Native, Indigenous individuals, children, and families.

All childbearing people who use cannabis during pregnancy deserve evidence based information, support, and care in their consumption and all families should have the option of choosing medical cannabis to support them during pregnancy, childbirth, and postpartum.

Methods of Harm Reduction

Cannabis substitution can be an effective harm reduction method for expectant people who are unable or unwilling to stop using tobacco, alcohol or other drugs, or who are not interested in using other prescribed medications at all.

Prior to consuming cannabis, if you are using other drugs, over-the-counter or prescribed, it is especially important to check for any possible drug interactions. Cannabinoids bind to the same receptors as most opioid medications and can make them work less effectively. Talk to your doctors to minimize any harm that may be associated with drug interactions.

Inhalation

- To reduce harm associated with smoking cannabis, always interpene your cannabis to make sure it has been properly grown and stored, free of bugs, mildew, and mold. Choosing quality flower also means insuring that your product is free of heavy metals and pesticides. If choosing to smoke, minimize the use of tobacco, spliffs, or cigar papers.
- Clean smoking items regularly, if using a bong, bowl, or pipe.
- Use hemp rolling papers, hemp wick, quality flower.
- Avoid mixing cannabis and tobacco.
- Minimize respiratory complications. Do you have a cough? — change method of consumption/check flower quality.
- Vaporize or steam instead of smoking. There are plenty options for dry-flower vapes, which I recommend over smoking. The Jamaican Steam Chalice is also a healthier alternative to smoking cannabis, which a sacred practice which involves heating the flower just enough to produce a steam without combusting plant material.
- Grow your own, choose quality flower, know your grower.

- Avoid using amounts that are large, or highly concentrated: Concentrates can contain heavy metals, and are often extracted using dangerous solvents. The Cannabis Doula does not recommend consuming concentrates during pregnancy if you are not a knowledgeable, experienced consumer.
- Ventilate and hydrate.

Ingestion

- Use caution when ingesting cannabis. Start low, and go slow. If you are new to edibles, start with the lowest possible dose (usually 5mg) and wait up to 24 hours before consuming a higher dose.
- Check for expiration date, sell-by date, batch number, and ingredients in all edible products to make sure you know exactly what you are consuming and when it was made.
- Keep in mind that when ingesting cannabis, THC metabolizes differently when it is passed through the liver for digestion and can affect us differently based on our unique metabolism and what we may have eaten before. It may take up to 3 hours before we notice any effects. Be mindful of this when consuming an edible at an event or social gathering.

Other Tips for Reducing Harm

- Incorporate holistic practices and alternatives to supplement use and boost your ECS naturally.
- Choose a legal, lab-tested source
- Track and manage cannabis consumption, using a cannabis journal
- Be Intentional: Check your Mental Health & Motivation
- Don't Drive High, or do anything that may trigger paranoia
- Consume a moderate amount with the appropriate consumption method.

Research on Cannabis & Pregnancy

There is conflicting research on whether or not cannabis is associated with preterm delivery, low birth weight, small for gestational age, decreased birth weight, newborn behavior issues, breastfeeding and infant motor development, birth defects including neural tube defect, gastroschisis, and frequency of use during adolescence.

There is no substantial evidence to suggest that cannabis is associated with any negative outcomes in pregnancy or while breastfeeding.

Research on cannabis use is limited due to moral/legal issues surrounding conducting research on pregnant / nursing people.

Current research does not take into account:

- CBD and other cannabinoids
- Methods of consumption
- Miscarriage
- Potency
- Why pregnant and breastfeeding women use
- Breastfeeding & cannabis use

Research Summary
Effects on exposed offspring of maternal marijuana use during pregnancy and breastfeeding

- No Substantial Evidence
(Cannabis is strongly associated with…):

- Moderate Evidence
(Cannabis is associated with): Decreased Growth, Decreased IQ scores in young children, Decreased cognitive function, attention problems

- Limited Evidence
(Cannabis may be associated with): Stillbirth, SIDS, Increased depression symptoms, Delinquent behavior, Isolated simple ventricular septal defects, Decreased academic ability

- Mixed Evidence
(There is conflicting research on whether or not cannabis is associated with): Preterm delivery, low birth weight, small for gestational age, decreased birth weight, newborn behavior issues, breastfeeding and infant motor development, birth defects including neural tube defect, gastroschisis, frequency of use during adolescence

- Insufficient Evidence

(No statements made): Psychosis Symptoms, Breastfeeding and SIDS, Initiation of future marijuana use

This research summary was taken from the Colorado Department of Health, and the extensive research they have gathered examining the risks of marijuana (THC) during pregnancy. They advise on many of the public health statements that are made across the country on cannabis and pregnancy. Taking into account the flaws and biases present in the research related to cannabis and pregnancy, it is important to consider all research as to influence methods of harm reduction.

Postpartum Cannabis Use

Cannabis can be safely used to support the mind, body, & spirit after childbirth. Cannabis is traditionally used to aid in postpartum healing remedies to relieve symptoms related to pain and to the following postpartum conditions:

Postpartum Mood Disorders
Postpartum Depression
OCD
PTSD
Baby Blues
Postpartum Rage
Anxiety
Hormone/Mood Imbalance

Cannabis & Breastfeeding

Cannabis preparations have traditionally been used to treat various breastfeeding concerns, however there has been very little research on cannabis & breastfeeding.

Mastitis, swelling/engorgement, clogged ducts, sore/cracked nipples can be relieved using various cannabis preparations.

It takes six days for THC to clear from breastmilk. THC is stored in fat; pumping and dumping is not useful with cannabis consumption as it is with alcohol. A fractional percentage of THC is transferred to the nursling of a mother who consumes while breastfeeding; effects are unknown. 2-AG is the primary cannabinoid found in breastmilk, and because phytocannabinoids perfectly mimic these molecules, cannabis is known to encourage the newborn feeding response.

Cannabis Postpartum preparations for increasing lactation:
Hemp seed rich diet, CBD oil, salves, topicals, infused oils, teas, and other holistic practices can help promote lactation. In some instances, especially for daily cannabis consumers, specific cannabis preparations (including poor quality cannabis) can actually decrease milk production. It is important to talk with a cannabis specialist if you are breastfeeding and consuming cannabis.

Cannabis Doula Care Consultation Common Question: If I smoke while breastfeeding, can my baby get high from drinking my milk?

Answer: From the way THC metabolizes in our body, it would be impossible, especially considering the small amount of THC found in the milk of mothers who consume cannabis daily. Infants and children have an ECS that is still developing, because of this children can often tolerate higher doses of THC without the same effect. Some doctors believe supporting the ECS in utero can have medicinal benefits, some do not! More research is needed to know for sure. If you do consume THC while breastfeeding, you can wait six days for the THC to longer be traceable in your breastmilk, or try consuming prior to breastfeeding.

CBD can be used by mothers who have concerns about THC. CBD oil, hemp seeds, and cannabis leaves can help alleviate soreness in breast and nippes as a result of breastfeeding. It can also help improve milk flow, clogged milk ducts, mastitis, etc. Juicing raw cannabis leaves can provide nourishment during the pregnancy and the postpartum period.

In some methods of consumption, cannabis can be used to inhibit milk flow, or it can be used to increase lactation. Use cannabis with consideration and caution while nursing.

Quality Cannabis Consumption

Source: In what country/state is the product grown? Indoor/outdoor? What is the strain used to produce this product? Where does it fall on the BLM-NLM spectrum? Is it grown naturally using organic processes?

Quality: How many milligrams of active cannabinoids (CBD, THC, THC-A, etc.)? Does the product contain? Total volume (milliliters) of the product? Is the product 3rd Party Tested for heavy metals, identity, and potency.

Why Interpening Cannabis is important: Visually inspect your flower. Most labs don't test for bugs, mold, or other defects in cannabis flower. Use Interpening! A strategy of using your senses to inspect cannabis, developed by Max Montrose at Trichome Institute. The Interpening Loop, Weed Wheel, and jewelers loupe are tools I recommend to help to ensure that the cannabis you are consuming is free of bugs, mold, is properly harvested and cured, properly trimmed with no seeds, and is safe to consume.

Cost: What is the cost per milligram? Do they offer financial assistance? Is there educational material / instruction to go with product?

Tracking & Managing Use

Record your daily use, the effects, and the properties of the cannabis product, to help you select the products and ratios that work best for you. Track your overall holistic wellness journey to make the most improvements in your wellness plan:

The Cannabis Diary & other cannabis journals or apps
Tracking physical, mental, emotional states prior to and after uses
Cannabis effects
Pain, allergies
Food, water intake
Exercise Sleep
Hormone Changes
Period tracking

Dosage Assistance

Experimenting can be helpful in finding your ideal dosage. Everyone is different, cannabis is unique, personalized medicine! Use the following to guide you in your consumption, not as medical advice.

By Product
- THC: 1mg per 20lb body weight
- CBD+THC: 1mg per 10lb body weight
- CBD: titrate up as needed
- Ratios (1:1, 10:1, 20:1) can help guide patients in finding the right dose

By Weight
- Under 150lbs: 2.5mg-5mg (in 24 hours)
- Up to 200lbs: 5mg-10mg
- 200lbs or more: 5mg-15mg

Be mindful of drug interactions if you are consuming opioids or other pharmaceutical drugs; high blood pressure, diabetes, anxiety, anti-depressants.

Cannabinoids taken in low/high doses can be ineffective; thresholds vary based on genetics, body weight, tolerance, and various other factors. Aim for an happy, effective "medium."

Suggested Dosage for CBD
Titrate up until desired results are achieved, then stop increasing dose. CBD dose may be lower if consumed with THC.

Day 1 and 2: 5mg
Day 3 and 4: 10 mg
Day 5 and 6: 15mg
Day 7 and 8: 20 mg
Day 9 and 10: 25 mg
Day 11 and 12: 30mg
Day 13 and 14: 35 mg

Dosage suggested by Healer (this a guideline, not medical advice)

Methods of Consumption

- Inhalation, smoking and vaporizing, are great for immediate relief. There are plenty of tools you can use to smoke or vape cannabis flower or concentrates, including water bongs, bowls, pipes, and fruit, or the steam chalice!

- Ingestibles, also referred to as edibles or gastrointestinal administration, such as capsules taken at bedtime or cannabis cooked and infused with food is ideal for supporting long term wellness.

- Topicals are great for everyday use, these include creams, salves, butters, soaks, bath bombs all of which aid in relaxation, relief, and support our body's largest organ--the skin.

- Submucosal Administration is great for women, children, and elderly cannabis consumers these methods are tinctures, taken under the tongue, hard candies, and rectal or vaginal suppositories.

- Transdermal patches and RSO are other ideal methods of consuming cannabis medicinally.

Cannabis Alternatives to Common Medications on Maternity Suites

Chronic Pain
Cannabis aids in both long term and immediate relief of inflammation, treating the source of pain and related symptoms + affective causes of pain.

Cannabis Profile:
- CBD-rich, THC, 1:1
- Broad Leaf to Medium Leaf
- Balanced is best for long term pain

Consumption Method:
- Topical
- Suppository

- Inhalation
- Transdermal
- Ingestible

Blood Pressure

Cannabis treats issues that indirectly cause high blood pressure: obesity, anxiety, and insomnia. Cannabis may speed up blood pressure & heart rate with initial use, then balance and regulate with long term use; relaxes blood vessels.

Cannabis Profile:
- Broad Leaf Dominant, High- THC
- CBD-rich

Consumption Method:
- Inhalation
- Sublingual
- Capsule
- Edible

Comfort Measures

Topical & internal cannabis applications provides relief for:

- Vaginal pain, dryness, discomfort after birth, during sex
- Sciata pain, and pain related to childbearing
- Hemorrhoids: Reduces swelling, burning, itching, soreness
- Soothes, protects, dry cracked skin and nipples (including diaper rash, eczema, psoriasis) and stretch marks

Cannabis can aid in immediate and long term comfort after childbirth and throughout the postpartum period.

Infection

Antimicrobial, Antibacterial, Antibiotic, Antiviral, Antifungal properties shown in cannabinoids: CBD, CBN, CBG, CBC, THC

Cannabinoids destroys harmful bacteria; more effectively than the strongest, least resistant antibiotic available: BV, Yeast infections, STDs.

Consumption Methods:
- Suppository
- Sublingual

Additional Support with Terpenes & Cannabinoids

Terpenes contribute to the smell, psychotropic effects, and medicinal benefits of cannabis, and are found within the plant's trichomes. Myrcene and pinene are the most abundant terpenes in cannabis. The medicinal benefits of the many terpenes in cannabis may act as an analgesic, antibacterial, anti-carcinogenic, bronchodilator, anti-convulsant, anti-fungal, and anxiolytic.

Cannabiniods are transporters, enhancers ,and regenerators within the ECS. There are three types of cannabinoids: endogenous cannabinoids that our bodies make naturally, phytocannabinoids found in cannabis, and man-made synthetic cannabinoids. The endogenous cannabinoid Anandamide is our internal bliss molecule (sanskirt, Ananda). It contributes to our sense of well-being and self-confidence during menstruation, childbirth; and is more abundant in the uterus than the brain! 2-AG is present in human breastmilk. THC perfectly mimics Anandamide.

Synthetic cannabinoids like the drugs Marinol, Sativex, etc. are FDA regulated and prescribed by doctors with some negative side effects being noted due to their isolated cannabinoids. The Cannabis Doula supports the use of phytocannabinoids like CBD and THC, and naturally boosting the body's production of endogenous cannabinoids.

Insomnia: Myrcene, linalool, terpinolene
Depression/ Mood: Limonene, pinene, B-Caryophyllene, CBD
Anxiety: Linalool, terpinolene, CBD
Energy: Limonene, eucalyptol
Anti-Inflammatory: B-Caryophyllene, CBGa, THCa, CBDa, CBCa, CBGVa, THCVa, CBDVa, THCV, CBD, THC, CBC, CBN
Cannabis works well with other herbs such as chamomile, ginger, turmeric, lavender, black cohosh, rosemary, and many others.

Cannabis preparations can also provide additional relief for:
Bloating, constipation, itching, allergies, headaches, and cannabis can also act as a laxative to support common postpartum discomforts.

Cannabis Infused Yoni Steam

Peristeam Hydrotherapy, or Yoni Steaming (vaginal steaming), is an ancient form of natural healing that has been used by people across cultures and around the world. Steaming is a gentle, relaxing, and rejuvenating therapy that involves sitting over a pot of steaming herbs, or water, using a stool or steam sauna. The healing steam softens and relaxes the cervix allowing the herbal properties to permeate the vagina, the uterus, healing and supporting the perineum. In fact, cannabis was often used in traditional and ancient practices of steaming, known as fumigation.

Steaming aids in healing and relief to common discomforts of the mind, body, and spirit, and can be practiced by people of all genders and ages. Incorporating cannabis in our steaming sessions, provides additional medicinal benefits, balance, and enlightenment.

Peristeaming is used to help treat a number of gynecological and emotional issues including but not limited to:

Regulating menstrual cycles, cramps, heavy flow, brown blood, endometriosis, PMS, ovarian cysts, fibroids, postpartum healing, vaginal infections such UTIs, yeast infections and BV, infertility, night sweats/hot flashes, bloating, painful sex, anxiety and nervousness, sleep challenges, stress, low libido.

Consult with a knowledgeable cannabis practitioner and yoni steam facilitator before incorporating cannabis into your vaginal steaming routine.

The Cannabis Doula provides Womb Steam Consultations, individual sessions, private events, and sacred group steaming sessions with cannabis. Learn more at www.thecannabisdoula.com.

Cannabis Infused Recipes

For the best infusions, use fresh cannabis that has been intentionally grown, using organic methods, free of pesticides, and other harmful chemicals, heavy metals, bugs, mold, and fungus. Learn to interpene your cannabis before consuming or infusing it. Cannabis is fat-soluble. It's medicinal components are extracted in fats, oils, alcohol, glycerin, and vinegar, which makes cannabis ideal for cooking and infusing!

Raw cannabis is not psychoactive. To activate the psychoactive components of cannabis, you have to decarboxylate your flower. Decarboxylation is a chemical reaction that involves carboxylic acids removing a carbon atom from a carbon chain; thus CBDa becomes CBD, THCa becomes THC, and so on for all the other cannabinoids. The acidic form has different medicinal properties. Decarboxylating can be done before or after infusing, by heating your cannabis flower. Cannabinoids activate at varying degrees. Depending on the cannabis and the effects you are hoping for, you'd want to make sure you are decarbing at the right temperature.

Cannabis Tincture

For the most potent tincture and for the most accurate dosing, we highly suggests using a concentrated form of cannabis (kief or RSO) and adding MCT oil, or vegetable glycerin, and using it sublingually.

RSO Tincture Method
- 1g of RSO=1000mg
- You can buy activated RSO, or make your own (see below).
- Start by heating your carrier oil or glycerin using a double boiler method. Use as much oil as you plan to bottle.
- Carefully, add RSO to the heated oil
- When all properties are melted and infused, remove the infusion from the heat. Let cool, then bottle and label with mg/ml and the date.

Kief Tincture Method
- Start by weighing the amount of cannabis kief you intend to use, 4 grams is a decent amount.
- Decarboxylate kief in the oven at 250 F for at least 40 mins.
- Use the amount of kief in grams divided by 2, to find the weight in fluid ounces of glycerin you need to use (20g of kief infuses into 10 fl oz of vegetable glycerin)
- Using a double-boiler method, heat glycerin oil to around 175 F
- Add decarboxylated kief to the glycerin carefully, stirring with a spoon
- Stir for 10-15mins, until mixture becomes syrupy
- Remove from heat, label, date, and store correctly

Alcohol Tincture Method
- If choosing to use alcohol for your tincture, I recommend the long-slow method of infusing food-grade grain alcohol with cannabis flower in a sealed jar for a few weeks, or using an infusion machine.
- For some people, alcohol can be slightly harsh for sublingual tinctures. You can also try a quick alcohol infusion by adding alcohol and herb in a jar and shaking vigorously for a few minutes, then straining the herb. Our recommended RSO and kief tincture methods are more potent, and safe for the whole family.

Cannabis-Infused Oil

There are plenty of methods for infusing cannabis into oil, and it can be used for cooking or for topicals. For a basic infusion, you can use a slow cooker, the double-boiler method, an infusion machine, a pressure cooker, or the classic 3-week infusion method. I recommend experimenting, and finding the method that is the most convenient for you. You can store infused oil in the refrigerator, or place in molds to make cannabutter. Use the oil of your choice, some are better for cooking, others are better for topical use. Our favorites are: olive oil, coconut oil, avocado oil, grapeseed oil, hemp oil, and sunflower oil.

Slow-Boil Infusion Method
- Add decarboxylated cannabis flower and oil in a sealed glass jar, stirring with a wooden spoon.
- Grinding your flower will allow for a more even infusion, but herbs

may be hard to strain
- Place sealed jar in a slow cooker, pressure cooker, or pot on the stove, with water. Allow the water to boil at a steady temperature for the herbs and oil to infuse
- The longer the infusion, the more potent. This method can be used for a 20min-12 hour infusion.
- Once your infusion is done, remove jar from the water and let cool
- Use cheese cloth to strain your infusion into a clean jar. You can strain more than once, if needed, to make sure all herbs are removed from the oil.
- Label, date, and store appropriately

Long-Slow Infusion Method

- Grind and decarboxylate cannabis flower and add to jar with oil
- Stir with wooden spoon, making sure all herbs are covered with oil
- Seal jar tightly, shake and store in a dark cool place
- Check on the infusion each day. Shaking, or opening the jar 1-3 times per day to insure no mold
- Let infuse for 3 weeks or more
- Strain infusion using cheesecloth into a clean jar.
- Label, date, and store appropriately

Infusion Machine Method (2-hour infusion)

- Grind and decarboxylate cannabis at the appropriate temp for 30 mins
- Add oil to Magical Butter Machine (2 cups or more for best results)
- Add cannabis flower to machine (7-14g minimum for best results)
- Select appropriate setting for infusion
- When machine is done infusing, let cool.
- Use cheesecloth to strain oil in glass, or air tight jars.
- Label, date, and store appropriately

Rick Simpson Oil (RSO)

RSO is a full extract cannabis oil, named after Rick Simpson who used the oil to treat his skin cancer. To make your own RSO, which is recommended, requires specific safety instructions, and lot of cannabis flower. RSO can be used to treat a number of life threatening conditions. This is one of the more potent forms of cannabis medicine.

To learn to make RSO, The Cannabis Doula recommends learning from Rick Simpson himself: https://cannabiscure.info/rso-cannabis-oil/

• Run For The Cure - The Rick Simpson Story: https://m.youtube.com/watch?v=zDJX7GqsQoA

• Rick Simpson & RSO Dosage Information: https://phoenixtears.ca/dosage-information/

Cannabis-Infused Honey

Infused honey is great for making cannabis infused tea, drinks, desserts, dips, dressings, and more. Infused honey sticks can also be used during birth. Both quality honey, and cannabis, are necessary.

Option One
• Combine dry, decarboxylated cannabis and organic honey in a jar
• Use wood spoon to stir and add more honey to the top of jar
• Let concoction infuse in an air tight container, for at least 5 days, making sure the herbs are completely covered flipping the jar each day, if necessary.
• Strain herbs using cheesecloth, and enjoy

Option Two
• Using the double-boiler method, combine dry, decarboxylated cannabis flower or concentrate and honey
• Allow concoction to heat and mix for 20-30 mins, strain flower and let cool (do not boil)

The ABCs of Herbal Remedies
for Pregnancy, Childbirth, & Postpartum

Anxiety: Hot bath/ Massage with bergamot, chamomile, geranium, lavender, Melissa, orange , or sandalwood essential oils + carrier oil. Catnip, Chamomile, Mint, fennel tea help to calm nerves

Breast engorgement: geranium, or peppermint essential oil cold compress. The leaves of green cabbage leaf along with small amount of hot waster, mashed together, let cool, apply mash to breast for 20-30mins. Warm compress of parsley or comfrey, apply to breast.

Discomfort in Birth: Motherwort tincture (5-10 drops in water, every hour). skullcap infusion or one teaspoon of tincture in water. St. John's wort infusion or 20-30 drops of tincture in water. Black cohosh root tincture in half-teaspoon doses. Plaque flower tea, tincture or capsule. Basil and gotu kola teas and sage compresses (used in Ayuverdic medicine.) Massage with clary sage, jasmine, lavender, nutmeg, rose or ylang-ylang essential oil + carrier oil. Catnip tea to coordinate contractions and ease pressure/discomfort.

Calm Nerves: Mint, Chamomile, Catnip, Fennel Tea (see Anxiety)

Colic: Fennel, Catnip, Chamomile, Calendula tea, massage

Constipation: Dandelion, marshmallow tea (leaves), steep and drink daily

Cystitis: corn silk thread, horsetail, or marshmallow tea

Easy Birth: Massage with Jasmine and lavender essential oil + carrier oil, or diffuse

Exhaustion in Birth: Infusion of fresh ginger root, raspberry leaf tea, and honey (don't use ginger if nearing birth, or for the first hour post-partum), infusion of rosemary tea, or tincture of blue cohosh root.

Gas: peppermint, chamomile, ginger tea

Headache: Fill sock with rice, lavender, rosemary, cloves. Warm sock in microwave, chill in freezer, apply to forehead.

Heartburn: Teas of ginger, Iceland moss, lemon balm, chamomile, marshmallow, meadowsweet, peppermint, spearmint

Hemorrhoids: Geranium, chamomile, and lavender. Massage essential oil + carrier oil on rectal area as needed. Pilewort cream combined with equal quantity of comfrey cream, or soak in a sitz bath of echinacea and comfrey tea.

Hemorrhage: Ergot tea (promotes contractions, use with support), Persimmon, Black Haw, Pepper tea

High Blood Pressure: Hawthorn and cramp bark tea

Insomnia: Nervine tea at bedtime. Massage Chamomile, lavender, candle wood, ylang-ylang essential oils + carrier oil, or diffuse.

Lactation: Massage Fennel, Jasmine, lemongrass essential oils + carrier oil. Teas of comfrey, dill, milk thistle, red clover alfalfa, nettles, fenugreek, hops, and vervain. Borage, blessed thistle, and wood betony as tea (for antidepressant + milk production). Fennel Seeds in tea, throughout day, chew and swallow (for milk production + infant colic). Bitter Melon tonic

Mood Changes: Herbal bath of roses, lavender, daisies or chamomile. Teas of raspberry leaf (with spearmint + peppermint). St. John's wort in capsule or tincture. Teas of vervain, lemon balm, lavender, lemon verbena leaf.

Morning Sickness: Anise, black horehound, chamomile, cinnamon bark, cloves, fennel, gentian, ginger root, Iceland moss, lavender, meadowsweet, raspberry leaf, rosemary, spearmint, or peppermint teas; Chew or sucking slippery elm tablets or candied ginger; red raspberry capsules or tonic. Lavender essential oil by inhalation or warm compress. Peach leaves

Muscle Aches: Fill sock with natural buckwheat, add clove, chamomile, and lavender. Warm in microwave, chill in freezer, apply to affected area. Soak Epson Salt.

Pain: (See Discomfort, and be mindful of language used in birthing!)

Perineum support (care/trauma/discomfort): Postpartum- calendula or comfrey, make tea, strain and add to sitz bath. Vitamin E oil, or calendula, comfrey, pilewort, St. John's wort, symphytum, hydrastis, and achillea creams or ointments can be topically applied to the perineum. Warm bath with lavender essential oil + carrier oil.

Postpartum Depression: Teas of chaste berry, motherwort, nettle, or raspberry leaf. Massage with uplifting essential oils like lemongrass, geranium, sweet basil, and lime + carrier oil. Bergamot, peppermint, ylang-ylang, or jasmine. Use as room freshener, diffuse, or add to bath with carrier oil.

Sleep Disturbances: Add cloves, mint, and rosemary to your pillow

Sore Nipples: Wash nipples with infusions of marigold or comfrey, expose to air and sunlight. Ointments of calendula, comfrey, plantain, St. John's wort, or yarrow heal cracked nipples and ease pain.

Swelling: Place cabbage leaves onto swollen area to draw out excess fluid. Soak swollen feet in Epsom salt. Apple cider vinegar compresses, or soak with ACV + water. Warm mustard oil massage. Warm bath with Eucalyptus essential oil. Cypress essential oil + carrier oil, massage area (also good for hemorrhoids, varicose veins, perineum support). Hydrate.

Threatened Miscarriage: Crampbark, or black haw bark taken in the form of decoction or drops, or tincture of chasteberry, or raspberry leaf tea

Umbilical Cord healing/hernia: Chamomile tea, Hawthornia: Hawthorn, litchi, and fennel seeds- slows, stops umbilical hernia growth. Shephards purse- reduce to paste and apply directly to hernia, externally to alleviate symptoms, internally to strengthen abdominal wall. Decoction of smartweed, lady's mantle, and walnut to soothe pain/discomfort, cover with bandage. Infusion of 1 cup of water and 1 oz of oak, yarrow, cypress, lady's mantle, and walnut.

Varicose veins: Tea, capsule, or tonic of blessed thistle. Lotions, compresses, and creams made from comfrey, marshmallow, marigold, plantain, yarrow, or hawthorn berries.

Water retention: Dandelion leaf, corn silk, or both, used in tea. Drink more water, dehydration can cause body to retain water.

Herbs to Avoid During Pregnancy

These herbs can induce abortion or miscarriages and should be avoided or used with caution during pregnancy: black cohosh, blue cohosh, celery root, pennyroyal, slippery elm douche, tansy, western red cedar, yarrow, rue, lovage, cotton root bark, Sweet flag, mistletoe, ginseng, golden seal, juniper berries, oil of sassafras, myrrh, southernwood, motherwort, angelica, marigold, bracken fern, golden ragwort and mugwort. Cannabis is not an abortifacient but was used along with these herbs to help mitigate the effects.

Essential Oils to Avoid During Pregnancy

Avoid the use of essential oils that can cause contractions during pregnancy such as cinnamon, clove, rosemary, and clary sage. The terpenes in cannabis are the essential oils of the plant. There has been no research on how terpenes in cannabis can impact pregnancy. I would not suggest using pure terpenes during pregnancy, unless for aromatherapy. Here are the oils you should avoid during pregnancy, or use with high regard and caution.

- Arnica (homeopathic is fine)
- Basil
- Birch (sweet)
- Bitter almond
- Boldo leaf
- Broom
- Buchu
- Calamus
- Camphor (brown or yellow)
- Cassia
- Chervil

- Cinnamon
- Clary sage
- Clove (bud, leaf or stem)
- Coriander
- Costus
- Davana
- Deertongue
- Elecampane
- Fennel
- Horseradish
- Hyssop
- Jaborandi leaf
- Juniper berry
- Melilotus
- Mugwort
- Mustard
- Nutmeg
- Origanum
- Parsley (large doses)
- Pennyroyal
- Pine (dwarf)
- Red cedar wood
- Rue
- Sage
- Santolina
- Sassafras
- Savin
- Savory (summer)
- Tansy
- Tarragon
- Thuja
- Thyme red (large doses)
- Tonka
- Wintergreen
- Wormwood, Worm Seed

Essential Oils to Use with Caution During Pregnancy

Caraway, Cedarwood, Chamomile, Clary Sage, Jasmine, Juniper, Lavender, Marjoram, Nutmeg, Peppermint, Rose, Rosemary

Disclaimer

For the best support with the use of herbs and essential oils, talk to your OB/midwife and consult with a traditional herbalist, or someone trained in the use of herbal remedies to support pregnancy and birth, Traditional Chinese Medicine, Ayuverda, or a cannabis specialist before incorporating cannabis and other herbal remedies during pregnancy, childbirth, and postpartum.

Statements made in this book regarding cannabis and other herbs have not been evaluated by the food and drug administration as the FDA does not evaluate or test herbs. This information has not been evaluated by the US Food and Drug Administration, nor has it gone through the rigorous double-blind studies required before a particular product can be deemed beneficial or potentially dangerous and prescribed in the treatment of any condition or disease.

The information presented here is provided for informational purposes only, and it is not meant to substitute medical advice or a diagnosis provided by your physician or other medical professional. Do not use this information to diagnose, treat or cure any illness or health condition. If you have, or suspect that you have a medical problem, contact your physician or health care provider. The products offered through The Cannabis Doula are not intended to treat, cure or prevent any illness or disease.

Use herbs as instructed by your care provider and always watch for any allergic reactions. Carefully read all product packaging and labels prior to consumption. Always consult your physician or health care provider before using any herbal products, especially if you have a medical problem or suspect a possible drug interaction.

The Cannabis Doula assumes no liability for any injury, illness, or adverse affects caused by the misuse and/or use of cannabis or the information, remedies, or products presented in this book, course, or website.

Talking to Doctors about Cannabis

Choose the right care provider
Build trust. Make sure you are comfortable with sharing that you consume cannabis. Most doctors, physicians, nurses etc. have not been taught about the Endocannabinoid System!

Find a doctor who specializes in cannabinoid medicine, supports or has knowledge of medical cannabis: online search, word-of-mouth, homeopathic/naturopathic doctors— like the Doctors Knox, who are a family of Black physicians trained in Endocannabinology.

Not all doctors can legally support cannabis as medicine because it is a Schedule 1 Drug, under hospital policy—even if they personally support it and use it. They may risk losing their licenses.

Some doctors work with pharmaceutical companies, and don't support or recommend herbal remedies, natural, traditional, holistic remedies— only prescribe Western treatments.

Ask questions.
Are they testing for THC without consent, forced consent, or coerced consent? What are their regulations regarding cannabis consumption during pregnancy? How do they support medical cannabis patients who become pregnant?

Birth Center/Hospital attitudes, discriminatory policies, illicit biases, and stigma surrounding cannabis use during pregnancy is very real, and does the most harm to cannabis consuming families.

Be knowledgeable.
Educating yourself on the medical cannabis and practicing safe cannabis consumption can help providers feel confident in supporting our decisions to consume medical cannabis during pregnancy. Schedule a Cannabis Doula Care Consultation with The Cannabis Doula to learn about cannabis use during pregnancy, safe consumption, and harm reduction to support a natural and holistic pregnancy and childbirth.

Cannabis & The Role of the Doula

There are many people who can support women and families in their cannabis consumption, but I believe that doulas specifically play a very important part in supporting families with cannabis. I may be a little biased. Doulas are awesome and, to me, truly represent the power of the divine feminine.

I was speaking to an older woman, a dispensary owner in DC, about cannabis use during pregnancy, and she shared with me her own personal experience as a woman giving birth in the 70s. She talked about how a doula first introduced her to the idea of cannabis use during pregnancy, and she and her partner agreed to try it. The only downside, she remembered it vividly as we all do our first births, was that everyone couldn't stop laughing during her birthing time! She said they were all laughing and she couldn't figure out what was so funny. Aside from their laughter, she described giving birth blissfully and in comfort, with the help of smoking cannabis. "I was so grateful for that doula, and I still am to this day!" We laughed.

A doula provides mental, emotional, and physical support to women and families during pregnancy, childbirth, and postpartum. Many traditional doulas have been trained in herbs and other natural, holistic remedies to support women. In fact, women who supported birthing people as traditional midwives and doulas used cannabis.

Women who used cannabis were often seen as witches and faced a lot of prosecution including death and the eradication of traditional midwives and healers in this country. The prohibition of cannabis is a reflection of this and the fear and propaganda that continues in our society. I became a doula after working at a medical cannabis cultivation center and becoming pregnant with my first son. It was hard. But it empowered me to advocate for women and families who did consume cannabis and has truly impacted my work as a doula; leading me down the path of reclaiming cannabis as a birth choice and health aid for women. Particularly for cannabis patients, doulas can act as cannabis caregivers.

Cannabis caregivers, depending on the state, support cannabis patients by crafting medicine, growing, or picking up products from dispensaries and educating clients on safe use. As a doula, I provide cannabis caregiver services in addition to other services, to women and families in my community. All doulas are unique and offer their own special wellness philosophies to the families they serve. I support families with cannabis and I encourage you, if you are a doula, to use this book, course, and future trainings as a stepping stone to learning more about cannabis.

There are plenty of cannabis certification programs available for birth professionals interested in learning to incorporate the herb in their practice. Be mindful, many doula organizations, doctors, hospitals and some communities are still unaware of the benefits and uses of cannabis use during pregnancy. Together, we can work to collectively advocate for families.

I'm bringing together doulas and birthworkers who advocate for families and their right to choose cannabis. If you are a doula and are interested in working collectively with The Cannabis Doula, contact me to learn more and get involved in all that we are planning for this year!

If you are currently pregnant and consuming cannabis, making sure your doula is informed and supportive of your choice is very important so that she can best advocate for you and your needs. If she is to be supporting you with cannabis preparations, it's also imperative that she is well-educated on cannabis, up-to-date and knowledgeable about research and methods to reduce harm are especially important to safely support a birthing person with cannabis.

Seven Steps Toward
Safe & Holistic Cannabis Consumption

1. Understanding the cannabis plant + how it interacts with your body (ECS), and research related to your condition
2. Examine the quality of your cannabis (Interpening!)
3. Analyze Social Implications: laws, doctor's attitude, stigma, family
4. Assess method of consumption & care needed to safely consume
5. Be intentional (mindful consumption)
6. Make an Informed Decision
7. Cultivate your Village + community of support!

Cannabis Legalization
as of November 2020

States & Territories with
Legal Adult-Use & Medical Marijuana Programs

Alaska
Arizona
California
Colorado
Illinois
Maine
Massachusetts
Michigan
Montana
Nevada
New Jersey
Oregon
South Dakota
Vermont
Washington
Washington, D.C.

Guam

States & Territories with
Medical Marijuana Programs Only

Arkansas
Connecticut
Delaware
Florida
Iowa
Hawaii
Louisiana
Maryland
Minnesota
Missouri

Mississippi
New Hampshire
New Mexico
New York
North Dakota
Ohio
Oklahoma
Pennsylvania
Rhode Island
Utah
Virginia
West Virgina

Puerto Rico
U.S. Virgin Islands

Countries with
Legal Adult-Use or Medical Marijuana Programs

Canada, Mexico, United States (Depends on State), Israel, Lesotho,
Ghana, Zimbabwe, Turkey, Chile, Brazil, Peru, Paraguay, Cayman
Islands, Belize, Costa Rica, Jamaica, Argentina
Colombia, Uruguay, Australia, New Zealand, India, Luxembourg,
Czech Republic, The Netherlands, Belgium

The Cannabis Doula Tip:
Know the laws in your state! Laws vary from state to state, country
to country. It is important to know the laws and attitudes regarding
hemp, marijuana use, THC and CBD.

The Cannabis Doula
Practitioner Training
Coming Spring 2021

A holistic cannabis doula workshop and training for trained and certified doulas to learn and support women, birthing people, and families who consume cannabis. This is a cannabis caregiver training centering the needs of women, birthing people, and families during the childbearing years. The virtual training will feature live virtual sessions, access to online cannabis education, and demonstrations of various preparations and remedies, including tips to grow cannabis medicine for others.

Holistic Cannabis Doula Practitioner Training participants will learn about cannabis use during pregnancy, childbirth, and postpartum, cannabis to support family wellness daily use, and preventative care. Participants will learn how to prepare cannabis preparations, how to interpene cannabis, consult with birthing families, and support conversations toward shattering cannabis stigma for the families they serve. Registration for the 6-month mentorship and training program is set to open in the winter of 2020.

Upon successful completion of the program, doulas will be Certified Cannabis Doulas, and receive three additional certificates in cannabis. To learn more, visit www.thecannabisdoula.org.

Shatter The Stigma with
The Cannabis Doula
Fundraising Campaign

The goal of this campaign is to provide communities most affected by the war on drugs and cannabis prohibition access to family-centered cannabis education, cannabis cultivation, & holistic services to minimize harm & stigma related to our cannabis use. We are raising $30,000 in capital for a space to house our educational programs, services, and trainings.

Our Mission

The mission of The Cannabis Doula is to support and advocate for women and families who choose to consume cannabis by providing femme and family-centered cannabis education, workshops, events, and a range of holistic birth doula services, culturally-competent childbirth education, and professional cannabis caregiver services.

Cannabis has been used to support women and families, especially for reproductive health and womb wellness, since the earliest known uses of the cannabis plant. Due to stigma, shame, and racial injustice, cannabis was outlawed and communities who have traditionally used cannabis have been criminalized, our families have been torn apart, and our communities were ravaged by the war on drugs—the lasting trauma, anxiety, depression, post-traumatic stress is still untreated in many victims and their families.

As medical cannabis use is being legalized all over the country, and globally, The Cannabis Doula™ seeks to mobilize women, especially women of color, to reclaim our ancient and traditional use of the cannabis plant; free of stigma, propaganda, and misinformation.

Our global mission is to reclaim and reconnect people of the African diaspora with cannabis, a plant that was spread all over the world, largely by our ancestors who were victims of the Trans-Atlantic Slave Trade. Our native and indigenous use and cultivation of hemp, as well as our instinctual knowledge and expertise of the cannabis plant, has survived tremendous hardship, and unsurmountable odds. Our belief is that we must collectively heal to overcome these grave injustices, and Shatter the Stigma related to our cannabis use— in order to learn, grow, and evolve as holistic, and knowledgeable cannabis consumers; turning poison into medicine.

Our Reach

Since launching The Cannabis Doula™ in 2018, we have had the tremendous honor of supporting women and families, both nationally and internationally, from DC to LA to Puerto Rico, and in places like Canada, Mexico, and the Netherlands. Through social media, consultations, classes, workshops and events, and numerous podcasts interviews, we've empowered women to address the stigma in their lives and implement holistic, safe cannabis use into their health and wellness regimes, and to support their individual families and unique communities.

It Takes A Village...
To Cultivate Cannabis.

As the cannabis industry continues to bloom, people of the African diaspora are continuously being left out, and social equity programs are failing. We are urging all communities to join our village and support our efforts to raise capital to further advocate for women's reproductive right to choose medical cannabis, safe access to quality cannabis for birthing families, and the woman-centered education, harm reduction, and care necessary for families to make informed decisions on cannabis.

To date, The Cannabis Doula™ has run completely on donations of members, people in our community and networks, and has largely been self-funded. As a small, Black, woman-owned, cannabis-centered company, we have not had access to business grants, or loans, or any other financial assistance due widely to injustice and ongoing cannabis censorship online which profoundly limits advertisements and marketing, and even education. We rely on word-of-mouth, provider and community referrals, and women sharing their experiences with cannabis during pregnancy through postpartum—which is exactly why we need your help to Shatter the Stigma!

By donating to our campaign, or in simply telling your story of how cannabis use has impacted your life as a birthing person—you can help expand the reach of The Cannabis Doula™ and help us fulfill our mission of providing woman-centered cannabis education, care, and support to families who need it most, across countries, communities, and cultures.

Fund Our Campaign; Support Our Village:

All funds donated to the Shatter the Stigma Campaign will be used in the following areas.

- To train and educate more women, mothers, doulas and cannabis caregivers to work collectively in support of cannabis choosing families
- To establish our headquarters and community wellness space to host our cannabis centered educational events, classes, retreats and services, including a child-care space and outdoor garden
- To invest in tech, supplies and material needed for the facilitation of our comprehensive childbirth education courses, our Holistic Cannabis Consumption: Pregnancy, Childbirth, and Postpartum course and workshop, and our Cannabis & Family Wellness class; and to make these courses, workshops and events affordable and accessible to all.
- To apply for cultivation licenses and permits necessary for home cultivation of medical cannabis, and the supply and equipment needed for our indoor and outdoor grow operations
- To globally empower, educate, and equip all women, centering women of color, on safe cannabis use, proper grow methods, and skills needed for supporting the unique needs of their communities

To donate and Shatter the Stigma, visit www.thecannabisdoula.org/donate, or email info@thecannabisdoula.com to partner or sponsor an event, training, or workshop.

Meet Melanin Ajé | The Cannabis Doula™

Thank you for joining me on this journey! I was called to birthwork after becoming pregnant while working at a licensed medical cannabis cultivation center in 2015. Facing stigma and discrimination, I began supporting and educating women and families who consume cannabis, especially during pregnancy, childbirth, and postpartum. In 2016, I started my journey as an independent birth doula and childbirth educator, training with DONA and Lamaze International, and certifying as a Hypnobabies® Hypno-Doula, a comprehensive medical-grade childbirth hypnosis program that supports families in having a painless, joyful birthing experience.

As a doula, I've studied traditional and holistic birth practices, holding certifications in Natural Holistic Remedies and Herbs and Nutrition in the Southern Tradition for Pregnancy and Postpartum. With a Bachelor of Science in Family and Child Studies with an emphasis in Family Social Services from Northern Illinois University, I've had the pleasure of serving and educating families in a variety of capacities through my business Happy Brown Baby LLC, where I offer family support services, doula services and a variety of family-centered educational support, centering Black women and families.

I am committed to learning and educating our communities about holistic cannabis consumption and reclaiming traditional birth practices through The Cannabis Doula courses, workshops, and events. I am a Certified Professional Interpener (cannabis sommelier), studying the art and science of cannabis, a certified cannabis consultant and educator, with several certifications from leading cannabis education platforms such as Green Flower, Cannabis Training University, Trichome Institute, Healer, and the American Journal of Endocannabinoid Medicine.

I'm a full-time mama of two happy, healthy toddlers combining my love and knowledge of cannabis with my drive to support and advocate for the health and wellness of women and families. Join me in reclaiming cannabis and let's Shatter the Stigma!

CPSIA information can be obtained
at www.ICGtesting.com
Printed in the USA
LVHW110718090421
683977LV00006B/129

9 780578 805399